Physician
Non Grata

Physician
Non Grata

*A Survival Guide for Clinicians Around
Poor Communication, Boundary Issues,
and Disruptive Behavior*

RYAN BAYLEY, MD

Distributed internationally via Amazon KDP services.

Physician Non Grata: A survival guide for clinicians around poor communication, boundary issues, and disruptive behavior / by Ryan Bayley.
ISBN 979-8-9877630-0-1 (pbk. : alk paper)
ISBN 979-8-9877630-1-8 (epub)

First printing, 2023

Pyriscent Coaching Press
1289 Fordham Blvd, Suite #205
Chapel Hill, NC 27514
Solvingcareers.com

For my wife India, and my daughters Ilaria, Hero, and Petra

CONTENTS

CHAPTER ONE

"My Good Name"

A cautionary tale

Mike was a vascular surgeon who had been in practice almost 20 years. The last twelve of those had been spent in a thriving private practice group operating out of a mid-size suburban hospital. He was well respected, very good at what he did, and, as far as he knew, well liked throughout the hospital.

One day the head of his practice group, Tony, poked his head into the OR during the last case of the day. He asked Mike when he would be done and could they meet in his office afterward. They agreed to meet at 4pm. Mike thought nothing of this - such impromptu meetings were common.

At 4pm Mike went to Tony's office. As he entered, he was surprised to also see Julia, who was one of the cardiologists and the Chief of Staff. Tony motioned for Mike to sit down and began by stating, "Mike, we've had a complaint."

Immediately, Mike's thoughts went to the Johnson case from last week. That case was a train wreck from start to finish. Both he and the PA surgical assist struggled throughout. The procedure could not be completed as planned and a less desirable alternative was performed. Although this had been discussed with the family ahead of time, they were still quite unhappy. Furthermore, the patient's post-op course was complicated - there were ventilator issues.

Ultimately, the patient was transferred to a tertiary care center and fortunately, last Mike heard, was slowly improving.

Already knowing the answer, Mike asked, "Which patient?"

"Actually, it's not from a patient, but from a staff member," Tony replied.

Mike's jaw dropped. He racked his brain for any friction-filled interaction over the last few weeks, and could not think of anything.

"From who?" he asked.

At this point Julia stepped in, "When we have a complaint like this we have a process to look into what happened to see if it's even valid. Until we do that, we can not discuss details, including who the complainant is because they have a right to confidentiality. As it is Thursday, we will put you on administrative leave for tomorrow which will give us through the weekend to talk to everyone. Then we will meet on Monday to clear this up."

Administrative leave?

Mike's thoughts raced between, "What the hell is going on?" and, "What am I going to do about tomorrow's patients?"

Tony could see the look on Mike's face. "Mike, it's just HR's standard process. I am sure this is a simple misunderstanding. We just need a day or two to work through it." He reiterated, "It is a standardized process."

Speechless, Mike realized there was really no choice in the matter, nor any further detail to be gleaned from this meeting.

Later, as he walked out to his car, he wondered how he was going to explain to his wife that he suddenly had tomorrow off.

———————

Initially, Mike spent the weekend alternating between feeling bewildered and guilty. Although he did not know what he was guilty of, he felt genuinely bad that someone had been so upset by something he had said or done. Certainly, he hadn't meant it. He wasn't that kind of physician.

But it wasn't long before that concern and bewilderment became frustration.

"This is ridiculous!" he thought. "I deserve to know what is going on."

So on Saturday he called in a few favors - after all, you don't work somewhere for twelve years without making a few friends. Pretty soon, he was able to piece together the basics.

The complaint did in fact have to do with the train wreck of a case from last week - but it was actually the surgical assist PA Samantha who made the complaint. Samantha was a relatively new PA. She had been with the hospital about six months. She was very competent and Mike thought they had a collegial relationship.

Apparently Samantha stated that Mike's behavior in the OR during the case was "abrasive and intimidating," and that it was not the first time. She also felt that his comments to her after the case were paternalistic and condescending, embarrassing her in front of colleagues as if he was shifting some of the blame to her. Furthermore, he put his hand on her lower back while standing very close to her making her physically uncomfortable, and this too was not the first time.

Mike was actually reassured when he learned all of this. "This could not be further from the truth!" he thought.

Yes, when the case started to go badly, he did speak more directly to everyone in the OR. But this was necessary for the safety of the patient and certainly wasn't personal. Things just needed to happen quickly and he needed everyone to be at their best.

And after the case in the PACU he saw Samantha was indeed upset, almost tearful. So he approached her. Standing next to her he tried to reassure her that this was a difficult case especially given her level of experience and that she would learn and grow from it. It was meant to be encouraging. He did not recall specifically touching her, although it was not unlike him to put a hand on someone to provide reassurance.

Mike spent the rest of the weekend mounting his defense. He practiced in his mind many times exactly how he would describe his perspective and intent. He also made a list of the many people in the OR and the PACU who he would call on if needed to corroborate his version of events. He was almost excited for Monday's meeting as an opportunity for vindication and, more importantly, to put this rapidly behind him.

————————

At Monday's meeting there were familiar faces. Tony, the head of his group, and Julia, the Chief of Staff, were present. There was also someone who he did not recognize who introduced herself as Linda, the hospital's lawyer.

Julia took the lead and explained the nature of the complaint, which matched the information Mike had already heard through the grapevine. She also stated they spoke to other people present, and felt the complaint had merit. The medical executive committee had concerns that Mike's communication in the OR was not conducive to optimum teamwork, and that his comments and physical actions presented boundary issues.

All of a sudden, it occurred to Mike that this was not the due process meeting that he was expecting. Rather, it all started to seem more like a *fait accompli*. He did interject, and argue his version of events noting multiple witnesses that should be called that would support him, but it didn't seem to matter.

Before he knew it, he had a piece of paper in front of him describing a voluntary "Performance Improvement Plan" focused on communication and boundaries. A quick glance over it revealed phrases like "zero tolerance" and "Physician Health Program." It seemed like a bunch of HR terminology. Mike's practice partner Tony reassured him that, while voluntary, the Performance Improvement Plan was the the quickest way to be able to resume clinical activity and to deal with this *"informally."* Mike did not like the way Tony kept emphasizing the word *"informally."* If this wasn't formal, what was?

Ultimately, Mike weighed his options. Reading between the lines it seemed like he had two choices. Go along with the plan or disagree. To disagree would seemingly trigger some type of more formal process, during which it seems he might not have active privileges.

Reluctantly, he signed. After all, what was he going to do, cancel all of this week's OR cases?

Does any of this sound familiar?

If you are reading this it is likely because you have experienced a similar process, or you work with those who have. If you have lived this yourself then perhaps the details of your story are different, but I am willing to bet that there are many elements of Mike's story that resonate. In my work, I hear a similar story almost every week from all types of clinicians.

I am also willing to bet that, like Mike, you did not *intentionally* mean to negatively impact someone with your speech or actions. After all, at some point you committed to "First, do no harm." So when an administrative review or disciplinary process concludes that your behavior was problematic, it is common to experience a wide range of challenging emotions.

For some that I work with, those emotions are guilt and embarrassment that another person was upset by something that they did. For others, anger and resentment are the dominant reaction. They feel that because their *intent* was not sinister, that they should not be blamed. Still others I work with do not even see how their behavior was problematic. For them, the whole process appears overblown and unjust. It is also not uncommon for clinicians I work with to vacillate between all of these feelings.

While these emotions are all predictable, they are not necessarily helpful in the big picture. When you fixate on your intent, for example, you can get so wrapped up in your own emotional experience and how you are going to salvage "your good name" that you neglect the other half of the equation - your impact. You forget that at the end of the day, another person felt your behavior was unacceptable, and, upon review, your peers agreed.

This is why you need this book

Until you can fully understand why someone found your speech or actions problematic, and why others agreed, you are at high risk of repeating the behavior and finding yourself in this situation again. You can often survive one such incident professionally, but rarely two. This is a real threat to your ability to continue to practice medicine.

So while you may stay awake at night worrying about the classic specters of malpractice, CMS violations, or personal disability, the reality is that it is events like Mike's that are far more likely to end your career. Unfortunately, no one has ever taught us how to navigate these treacherous waters and come out better for it on the other side. I don't know about you, but this scenario was never discussed when I was in medical school. That is the impetus for writing this book.

Having spent years as an executive coach and advocate for physicians, I have worked with many of your colleagues navigating similar waters. I have seen the same patterns play out over and over. I have seen the same blind spots and lack of knowledge make a bad situation worse. I have watched clinicians dig their heels in, and be dismissive and fixated on "the system," only to make the same mistake again with even bigger consequences.

This book is thus an amalgamation of everything I have learned working with physicians accused of poor communication, boundary issues, or disruptive behavior. Ultimately, the goal is to provide you with a road map for achieving a good outcome from this event. This includes being able to continue to practice medicine. It includes avoiding, or at least minimizing, a medical board action or National Provider Database report that will follow you for years. Most importantly, a good outcome means completely understanding what was problematic about what you said or did, and learning new skills and mindsets so that your future behavior is above reproach.

To that end, we start the next chapter by exploring exactly how an administrative action or disciplinary process unfolds. It is often a months- to years-long process involving a whole host of mechanisms and organizations that you will have to navigate. It is essential that you quickly orient yourself to this system.

Next, we will briefly touch upon the immediate actions you should take to avoid further damage in the short run.

Lastly, we will focus on all of the ways our behavior create problems for ourselves and others in today's healthcare environment. Whether you were uncivil to a colleague, made an inappropriate joke, violated someone's personal space, were perceived as hostile in an email, or advocated to the point where you were labeled as disruptive, this book will help you understand what went wrong, your role in that wrong, and how to do things differently in the future.

Regardless of where you are in the process, there is information contained in this book that can help you. Read carefully and with an open mind and it might just save your career.

CHAPTER TWO

Kafka-esque

Navigating what happens next

Kaf • ka • esque *(käf - kə - ˈesk)*
Of, relating to, or suggestive of Franz Kafka or his writings - especially having a nightmarishly complex, bizarre, or illogical quality.

When Mike signed his Performance Improvement Plan, he thought that was the end. But in reality, it was the beginning of an almost year-long process of increased scrutiny, unclear endpoints, and a lot of time and money spent.

For Mike, the process first took on a kafka-esque nature when he did not experience the due process he imagined would be afforded to him in the initial accusation. Like most physicians who hear a complaint has been made, he assumed there would be an almost trial-like process, where he would be afforded an assumption of innocence until proven guilty beyond a reasonable doubt. He assumed he would hear directly from the complainant and be able to rebut. He assumed the hospital's process would be open and transparent. He assumed he would be allowed, indeed required, to present a defense.

The problem is that these assumptions are grounded in a gross misunderstanding of the legal framework that governs our ability to practice medicine.

For starters, the Medical Board grants you the *privilege* to practice medicine within your state (not the *right* to practice medicine). Similarly, an organization grants you hospital *privileges* to practice within their facility (not hospital *rights*). Now while this difference between rights and privileges may seem semantic, it is actually quite profound.

Generally these types of privileges fall under the paradigm of administrative law. This means that your "case," so to speak, won't be decided in a trial or through arbitration as we see it done on TV. Rather, the privilege-granting organization itself will be judge, jury, and executioner. Administrative law grants broad powers of self-governance. As such, it will be up to the organization as to what processes it follows, and its decisions are rarely subject to some higher authority or oversight process. Appeals processes are limited or, on a practical level, non-existent (for reasons we will soon discuss).

This results in two hard truths

Truth #1 - There is no presumption of innocence. Medical Executive Committees exist to protect the patients and hospital employees from *you*. Medical Boards exist to protect the public from *you*. If a complainant says that you communicated poorly, had a bad attitude, created a hostile work environment, violated a personal boundary, made an inappropriate joke, etc, you will have a hard time convincing these entities otherwise. The complainant's perception is given tremendous weight, and unless you have audio or videotape it is going to be hard to argue against perception.

Truth #2 - Whatever these entities decide is final. If one of these entities concludes that you were in the wrong, then you were in the wrong. If you wish to retain your privileges with that entity, you will have to complete whatever corrective process they recommend.

These two truths can be tough pills to swallow. But the sooner you wrap your mind around them, the sooner you can move in a meaningful direction. I have seen too many physicians get headstuck, unable to accept the fundamental reality of how these organizations operate.

So what happens next?

Your medical board / medical executive committee / employer has decided that you have spoken or acted poorly. Now what?

What happens next can vary widely, but it usually involves interacting with one or more of the following:

- Performance Improvement Plan (PIP)
- Workplace Monitor
- Physician Health Program (PHP)
- Physician Assessment Professional (or Program)
- State Medical Board
- Physician-specific classes or treatment programs
- Physician coach or therapist

The rest of this chapter will be spent exploring each of these elements and how they might be used in a given physician's case.

Performance Improvement Plan

Performance Improvement Plan (PIP) is a human resources euphemism for WRITTEN WARNING, and in most cases, FINAL WRITTEN WARNING. It is usually generated by your organization, or sometimes by a third party brought in to consult on the issue (such as a Physician Health Program (PHP) - see below).

A well-written PIP should:

- Clearly identify the performance / behavior that needs improving.
- Provide specific examples and reasoning.
- Outline the expected standard going forward.
- Identify any training or support to be provided (or mandated) to achieve this change.
- Specify how this will be monitored, by who, and on what schedule
- Have a mechanism for on-going and timely feedback DIRECTLY TO YOU
- Have an end point
- Explain what will (or won't) change upon completion of the PIP, as well as if you don't complete the PIP

The problem with many PIPs, however, is that they do not address the points above. It is not uncommon that the person writing the plan has either never written one or never received guidance on how to write a good one. Without malicious intent, PIPs can often be vague, leave out pertinent information, and set you up for ambiguity or failure.

As such, it is imperative that ask for clarity on all the above points before signing. Once signed, this document serves as the measuring stick of your behavior going forward. It is also the main document the organization will use to defend its decision to revoke your privileges and/or terminate your employment in the future. You should understand it and be crystal clear about its content.

Workplace Monitor

Many PIPs will designate a Workplace Monitor. This is generally a senior peer whose role is to observe your demeanor, appearance, and interactions in the workplace. Ideally this is someone you work with on a regular basis and, to the extent possible, have a limited conflict of interest with. They are meant to be a stable and trustworthy resource for you, as well as a watchful and diligent monitor for the organization.

If that all sounds contradictory or impossible, it is. First, as physicians, we don't really work with other physicians. Yes, there are other physicians around, but we don't actually work together that often. Whoever is chosen for this role will have a hard time *directly* observing your demeanor and behavior on a frequent basis. They will have to rely on word of mouth and second-hand accounts.

Second, who is your peer that you work with frequently who is not going to have some glaring conflict of interest? Not surprisingly, the Workplace Monitor is often in a very difficult position. It is certainly not a job that I would want.

Regardless, if a Workplace Monitor is used in your case, you need to clarify many important points just as you did with the PIP above. Who is the monitor? How will they observe you? What are their expectations and reporting criteria? How often will you meet? Can you have a confidential conversation with them about a challenge, or is it not confidential?

Also, like the person writing the PIP, the person chosen as Workplace Monitor has likely never done it before and likely will be given little guidance from the organization. It is your right to seek clarity and ask the Workplace Monitor to seek clarity at the beginning of the process to hopefully avoid a problem later.

Physician Health Program (PHP)

Physician Health Programs (PHPs) are generally described as "a confidential resource for physicians (and other licensed healthcare professionals and trainees) who suffer from addictive, psychiatric, medical, behavioral, or other potentially impairing conditions." Almost every state has a PHP. It is usually an independent non-profit organization, sometimes affiliated with, or even funded by, the state medical society.

PHPs historically functioned as a resource to help physicians recover from substance or alcohol abuse. The idea was to create a structure whereby a physician could seek help, enter recovery, and eventually continue to practice in a monitored way that preserved their career while keeping the public safe. Over time, most PHPs evolved to take on a larger array of challenges, including helping physicians with mood disorders, personality disorders, or neurocognitive disorders that impacted performance or behavior. Furthermore, many PHPs have expanded to serve advanced practitioners, dentists, pharmacists, and veterinarians.

Even more recently, burnout, poor emotional intelligence, interpersonal communications challenges, cultural conflicts, and boundary issues are now often considered the purview of PHPs as well.

Thus it is increasingly common that as part of a PIP or medical board investigation you will be referred to your state PHP. The referring organization will state that this is for your benefit, as PHPs can provide a much more comprehensive assessment and ideally not miss an underlying pathology or stressor that your organization (and perhaps even you) are not aware of. It is also to the benefit of the organization, as it makes them look extra diligent and thus provides legal cover if they ultimately revoke your privileges and fire you.

In my opinion, perhaps the most important benefit to you is that PHPs have the resources and experience to best support you in successfully moving forward. As alluded to above, when organizations write a PIP they are often very good at spelling out what they did not like about your behavior. Unfortunately, they are usually not so good at clearly articulating the behavior they want, and they are dismal at providing resources to support real change. This is because they simply do not know - they expect you to figure it out. Fortunately, PHPs generally have a wide array of assessments and resources such as physician coaches, therapists, and programs that they can recommend.

A quick head's up on what to expect from a PHP interaction:

Before moving on, it is important to give you a head's up as to what your PHP encounter will entail, as many physicians are often surprised. First, when you walk in you will probably be handed a cup to pee in for your drug test. Many physicians are taken aback by this. "I was sent here because a patient felt I was too cavalier during a breast exam, and you are treating me like an addict!"

You have to remember that historically the PHP's raison d'être is to identify and treat drug and alcohol addiction. Also, you have to think like a mental health clinician. Remember the DSM from your psychiatry rotation in medical school? You probably learned from it that you can't diagnose anything if a substance or alcohol use disorder is present. The assumption is always that if such a disorder is present, it is the driver of behavior. You can only deal with any remaining behavioral issues once that disorder is managed. Thus the PHP has to rule this out first.

Then, the focus shifts to DSM psychopathology. Do you have a mood disorder, personality disorder, or neurocognitive disorder that contributed to the events leading to the referral? You may feel that you do not, but sometimes you are the last to know. It can also make a big difference, perhaps even in your favor - consider the following example:

> *A third year resident was referred to the PHP for sexual harassment / boundary violations. Effectively, his program was going to fire him. While there were multiple incidents, the most egregious was his harassment of a nurse who he asked out repeatedly and gave gifts to over a period of six months. She always rebuffed him. In her mind she was crystal clear about her lack of interest, but the resident persisted. Eventually she reported it to her organization's HR hotline and the medical board.*

> *The PHP assessment quickly revealed the resident had a high-functioning autism spectrum disorder. He had often been thought of as "quirky" but no one had ever diagnosed his autism because he was such a high performer. When he would ask the nurse out for the coming weekend, and she would say no, he could not read between the lines or interpret her cold body language. He took her response literally and at face value, thinking she just meant no for this weekend (despite saying no for the 20th weekend in a row). If she had ever said to him, "I don't like you, and never will, and I will never say yes," he would have understood and stopped immediately. But of course she was never that blunt.*

> *Once his autism was understood, it put everything into a new perspective for his residency director who had written him off. A comprehensive plan was created to support the resident and work on social skills. He did eventually complete his training.*

Now again maybe you are certain you have no psychological disorders. Nonetheless, the PHP is going to assess for that. You will likely undergo a very extensive multi-hour interview process where they will ask you very personal questions beyond the scope of your professional practice. It is not uncommon for clinicians I have worked with to be frustrated by the broad focus and personal nature of these interviews - "I am here because a colleague did not like my opinion on *Blue Lives Matter,* not because I have a *real* problem!"

Thus, from the clinician's perspective, the scope of the interaction with the PHP can seem quite broad - but there is an important logic to it. PHPs need a systematic process to assess and help *everyone* who walks through their door. This encompasses an incredibly wide range of provider types and issues - running the gamut from a public-endangering addiction to a politically-charged conversation that created workplace tension. As such, they apply a formulaic and comprehensive approach to every person, every time, regardless of the reason for referral and regardless of whether they were mandated or voluntarily self-referred.

So if you have not yet met with the PHP I hope these last few pages will help you know what to expect and help you better understand their role. If you've already been part of a PHP process, I hope these last few pages will help normalize that process, especially if you found it surprising.

Also, one last thing worth mentioning before we move on: if you work for a particularly large organization (a major academic system for example), you might be referred to an internal equivalent of the PHP. Some organizations have internal physician support programs that provide much the same function. If these programs are robust and physician-specific, they can be good.

Unfortunately, many large institutions instead refer physicians under a PIP to their Employee Assistance Program (EAP). These are highly variable in quality and often generally useless in terms of their ability to be helpful in physician-specific situations. Should you find yourself mandated to an EAP and underserved, you can always self-refer to a PHP or inform your employer about the existence of the PHP as an alternative. In reality, most organizations and physicians are not aware of their state PHP as a resource.

Physician Assessment Professional (or Program)

As we just discussed, most physicians who have an assessment performed have that assessment performed by their PHP, or their organization's internal equivalent. However, there are third-party assessors as well. Some of these are individual practitioners, usually with a mental health background, who have developed a niche working with physicians. There are also a handful of third-party assessment programs around the country that specialize in physicians.

These third-party assessments usually occur in one of three scenarios. First, a third-party may be used when a more niche, focused assessment is needed beyond the initial one. Take our example of the third-year resident with autism. By the end of his initial PHP evaluation, the person doing the assessment highly suspected that he was not some kind of sexual predator with a disregard for boundaries, but rather that an autism spectrum disorder might be at play. So at that point, the resident might be referred to a third-party who specializes in assessing neurocognitive disorders in high functioning professionals to ensure the correct diagnosis and treatment.

A second scenario where third-party resources may be used is in the case of smaller PHPs. Funding for PHPs varies tremendously, and thus some PHPs do very little assessment internally. Rather, they rely on a community of independent practitioners who they refer to. In these cases, the PHP functions more as a go between. When someone is sent or self-refers, the PHP triages and connects them with assessment resources.

A third scenario, and by far the one I have seen most commonly, is when a physician disagrees with the conclusions of an initial assessment and demands an independent evaluation. Usually at that point they are offered the option of obtaining a more comprehensive evaluation through an independent provider or physician assessment program (usually out of state).

It is important to note that in all of these scenarios you generally bear the cost when a third-party assessor is used. When the use of that third-party assessment is mandated (i.e. a stipulation of your PIP, for example), it may feel coercive because if you don't undergo the assessment, you may be perceived as non-compliant with your PIP. You have no choice in the expense.

It also makes appealing a decision a much less practical option, as we can see in the following example:

> John was reported to his organization after having a heated discussion regarding religion and abortion with a group of female medical students he was supervising. A PHP assessment was recommended as part of the internal review. The PHP concluded that John exhibited weak boundaries, poor perspective taking, and furthermore had trouble appreciating the significant power dynamic at play between students and attendings. The PHP recommended a two day professional boundaries course and for him to work with a physician coach for six months.

> John thought this was ridiculous and appealed. He was informed his only avenue for appeal was an independent assessment through a third-party physician assessment program. The closest one was in an adjacent state 8 hours away. Their assessment was a three day, six hour per day structured program. He would have to get the time off, travel, spend three nights in a hotel, and pay for the assessment at a cost of over $10,000 when all was said and done. He did it anyway because he was sure he would be vindicated.

> Two months later he received the comprehensive evaluation, which came to most of the same conclusions and recommendations that the PHP did.

This is not to say that third-party assessments are never worthwhile as an appeal mechanism. However, you have now been warned - these can rapidly become quite costly and they more often than not come to conclusions similar to the initial evaluation.

State Medical Board

State medical boards may become involved if the complaint against you is made directly to them, and not to your organization. Sometimes, the complainant just believes the medical board is the correct place. Or sometimes, the complainant doesn't trust their organization to really do anything about a complaint. When 20 nurses have called their organization's HR hotline 20 times over the last two years about a certain doctor who keeps making sexual innuendo and nothing has happened, eventually someone is going to go to the medical board.

Regardless of how it occurs, a complaint to the medical board represents greater jeopardy for you. Medical boards are tasked with protecting the public (i.e. patients) from bad medicine. This is the lens through which they view any complaint. They will look at the complaint and ask, "Is this a clinical care or poor judgement issue? Is there a technical competency problem? Did the physician disregard patient safety or violate a patient's trust? Is the physician committing medical fraud?" For the types of problems we are focusing on in this book, the answer to these questions as far as the medical board is concerned is generally "no." Once they reach that conclusion, they will usually refer the complaint to your organization and/or the PHP.

However, you are now on their radar and you likely now have an "open case." That is never a good thing. They will often keep tabs on the situation and request updates through your organization or PHP for months or, in some cases, years. Anything else that comes up in regards to you vis-a-vis the medical board will be looked at through a colored lens. It is a major strike against you moving forward.

Physician-specific classes / programs

At this point you have been assessed either by a PHP, internally at your organization, or by a third-party. Conclusions have been reached and recommendations made. One common recommendation is that you attend a class specifically for physicians that focuses on any deficiencies identified.

Such classes are run by many of the same third-party programs that do assessment work. Typical topics for these classes include professional boundaries, interpersonal communication, stress-management/burnout reduction, ethics, and documentation/record keeping. Historically these were 2 to 4 day, in-person courses. Again, this meant travel as well as significant cost for the course itself (often $1000-$2000 per day).

However, COVID did change the way many of these programs operate. Initially, all of the programs had to be cancelled as travel and in-person instruction was not possible. It took a while, but many programs did move to a virtual format.

As of the writing of this chapter, some programs have moved back to in-person instruction only, while others still have some virtual options. Personally, the physicians I know who have done these courses said the primary benefit was interacting with their peers *in person.* In an intimate and vulnerable way, this allowed participants to understand how their peers erred, got tripped up by their own blind spots, and how common themes pervade the wide-range of reasons to be referred to such a program - all leading to tremendous self-insight. To some extent, this efficacy is lost in the virtual world. Thus many programs have moved back to in-person formats. Regardless of format, these courses are often booked out months in advance as demand continues to steadily climb.

Therapist or Physician Coach

Another common recommendation is for you to work with a therapist or physician coach. This may be used as an adjunct to a course, to help keep you accountable and continue the work you started in the course. Other times it may be the only recommendation.

Whether you are recommended a therapist or a coach depends on many factors, including the nature of the challenge, the referring organization's comfort with each modality, and sometimes your preference may be considered as well.

When dealing with DSM diagnoses - i.e. a mood disorder (ex: depression or anxiety), a clinical personality disorder (ex: borderline personality), or a neuro-cognitive disorder (ex: OCD, ADHD, autism) then you must work with a therapist or psychiatrist. For skill building, such as it relates to interpersonal communication, boundaries, leadership/self-leadership, or time-management/workflow - these are increasingly the domain of coaches.

Sometimes because of these differences, people will say the focus of therapy is healing, whereas the focus of coaching is succeeding. Or they will say that therapy focuses on insight and understanding, whereas coaching focuses on goal creation and execution. These are all oversimplifications. There are therapists who practice very goal- and action-oriented types of therapy. And while coaching is not therapy, it can be very therapeutic.

Regardless of the recommendation, you should understand clearly what the recommender hopes you will get from the modality. You should also have your own goals. When a physician is referred to me for coaching I always ask them what they hope to achieve. When they reply, "I hope to show up once a month for an hour and satisfy this mandated recommendation from the PHP so that they will leave me alone," that is not an auspicious start. When they show up and say, "I hope to better understand what has happened, and what I can do differently to avoid this happening again," that is promising. When they say, "I want to learn skills and new ways of being to improve my workday and how others experience me at work," that is even better!

Now you know the lay of the land

You now have the 30,000 foot view of all of the major entities that play a role in administrative reviews and disciplinary processes. If you are well into your journey, you likely have encountered at least a few of them (and are probably asking where was this book a few months ago?). If you are just starting out on your journey, you are probably a little nervous.

Regardless, it is now more obvious why this process is experienced as kafka-esque. Multiple factors coalesce to make this time particularly disorienting and distressing for any clinician:

- Incorrect assumptions regarding how the initial complaint process will play out, which are the result of ignorance regarding administrative law, especially as it relates to due process
- Suddenly having to navigate formal processes and entities that you did not even know existed (PIPs, PHPs, etc)
- A slow, step-wise progression through a system were every evaluation or conversation seems to result in another referral or recommendation
- Nebulous expectations and evaluation processes from your group/employer from the beginning
- Lip service to participation being voluntary, when really it is mandatory if you wish to continue to practice
- A significant amount of cost in terms of time and money
- A process that is often still unfolding one to two years after the inciting event

And the system certainly has its critics, just search the internet.

But for all the critics there are many advocates, including many physicians who have benefited from the process. Advocates argue that without this system, most physicians would simply be fired or lose licensure. Ten years ago behavior that would have been ignored is now too high a risk for your organization to tolerate. These resources give the organization options, so to speak - a way of trying to salvage a situation where their hands would be otherwise tied.

Also, most administrators and clinicians who work in this system are sincere and highly motivated to help their peers. Many people who work for PHPs are in recovery themselves, for example. Many people who teach physician-specific classes on boundary issues and communication are physicians who temporarily or permanently lost licensure for the exact same reasons.

But I digress.

The point of all of this that I have just laid out is not to debate whether the system is "right" or "wrong." It is to tell you how it is - forewarned is forearmed. Now you understand all of the pieces and how they move on the board. Knowledge is power.

But what if you don't want to accept this? What if you adamantly refuse to play the game?

Usually at this point one of two ideas will pop into your head, **sue or quit**. So let us discuss each of those.

Can't I just sue my employer / the PHP / the Medical Board?

Of course you can! This is America! You can sue anyone for anything at any time.

Suing would appear to solve certain issues. For example, if you feel the process you have been put through lacked due process, was not transparent, was unfair - then it is a completely rational thought that suing and putting this all in front of a court would force due process, transparency, and objective judgement into the situation.

On a practical level, however, there are two caveats. First, this will take time, and second, there is no guarantee you will prevail.

In regards to time, legal action will take at least one to two years to reach a conclusion, and maybe even longer. In the meantime, everything gets put into suspended animation. If you try to work somewhere else during this time, that place will call your previous employer and be told something vague but ominous like "litigation is pending." Credentialing at other places may run into significant roadblocks, with many potential employers and insurers saying, "We can't wait to work with you, we just need to see how this plays out first." It may be harder than you think to find temporary employment (but not always impossible).

If your license was suspended or put in some type of probationary status, this is a bigger problem. It is highly unlikely that you will have a usable license until the case has run its course. Many physicians cannot tolerate this type of income disruption in addition to the significant cost of litigation.

Now of course if you were to prevail you may be able to make up for this with monetary damages. But that is a *big* if. Without going into too much legalese, it is important to understand that any time a clinician's right to practice is called into question, there are complex legal issues that come into play. These include property rights, liberty interests, the right to work, public safety, and the sanctity of peer review processes. For over one hundred years these often conflicting issues have been debated by courts when deciding both a clinician's ability to practice and the power of medical boards and hospital committees to regulate that ability.

As such, cases can have many different outcomes. More often that not, however, courts are reluctant to interfere with the decisions and self-governance of employers, hospital privilege committees, and medical boards. Even if a lawyer feels that your specific case is strong, he or she will be the first to tell you there are no guarantees that you will regain privileges, retain licensure, or be compensated sufficiently for lost wages and other damages.

But I am not a lawyer.

So please do not let this talk you out of pursuing legal recourse. Seek counsel, have these conversations. Just understand that legal action will not be a quick fix or a guaranteed win.

Fine. Then I will just quit - there are other fish in the sea.

NO MATTER WHAT YOU DO, DO NOT QUIT OR VOLUNTARILY SURRENDER PRIVILEGES IN AN ATTEMPT TO END A DISCIPLINARY / REVIEW PROCESS!

This is one of the most tragic errors I see, and many physicians make it before I even start working with them. The reason that this is such a problem is due to a little known rule regarding the National Provider Data Bank (NPDB). The rule states that organizations are required to report "a practitioner's surrender of, or failure to renew, privileges while under or to avoid investigation." Similarly, state medical boards are required to report "a dismissal or closure of a formal proceeding because the practitioner surrendered licensure or left jurisdiction."

So consider the following true story:

> *Felix was an independent orthopedic surgeon with privileges at three hospitals. Tonya, a CRNA, had been on leave for a few weeks. It was widely known that this was for a breast augmentation. When she returned, Felix made a comment to her in front of a few colleagues that "they did great work." He and Tonya had worked together and joked together many times in the OR, and she had been open with him about her upcoming procedure. Thus based on their previous interactions he thought this comment would be well received. Tonya was clearly flustered, and reported the event to her supervisor.*

> *Felix was notified and told this was being "looked into" especially given that he was about due to renew his privileges. The Medical Executive Committee would have to review it, possibly delaying his re-cert. He would likely have to appear before the committee at their next meeting.*

> *Even before this incident, Felix had already been thinking of not doing further cases at this hospital for various logistical reasons. As such, he decided to just not complete his renewal application and let his privileges lapse. It all just wasn't worth the hassle.*

> *Six months later, when applying for privileges for some additional locums work, he was denied. He was informed that the reason was due to his National Provider Data Base record, which now stated, "Voluntarily surrendered privileges while under investigation for sexual harassment."*

Unfortunately for Felix, such a line is really no less damaging than if it had said, "Privileges revoked following an investigation for sexual harassment that concluded allegations were founded." To future employers, privileges committees, recruiters, medical boards, and insurance companies, the type of statement on Felix's NPDB record is synonymous with guilt even though no guilt was proven. I have seen such statements make many physicians' lives very difficult.

It is also impossible to get such a statement removed, because it is factually correct. NPDB statements can be modified or voided if they are incorrect, or if the action is reversed on appeal or overturned by a court. But in this case, the statement is 100% accurate and there is nothing to appeal - Felix did not complete his bi-annual renewal application for privileges while under an administrative review process. The statement simply reflects the reporting requirement - which is to report that he *failed or chose not to* renew privileges while under investigation.

The irony is that often when physicians surrender privileges, quit, or move to try to end a disciplinary process, the result is often worse than if they had completed the process with a negative outcome. The NPDB only reports professional review actions that affect one's privileges for more than 30 days. So if our friend Felix above were found to be in the wrong regarding a boundary violation, clinically suspended for two weeks, and mandated to complete a 6 month PIP and a undergo a PHP evaluation, there is a good chance that would have never meet threshold criteria for an NPDB report.

With medical board actions the threshold for reporting is lower. They are required to report any actions that result from a formal proceeding. However, many of the situations this book is written for will result in a medical board taking an informal action, such as referring to a PHP, which is often considered a confidential referral and is not reported. PHPs also do not report directly to the NPDB.

Quitting or surrendering privileges while under scrutiny actually makes your organization's job too easy. It solves a major problem for them (i.e. the problem of investigating you), and they just make a report to the NPDB that states that you quit while under investigation for X or Y offense. They never have to prove the claims made against you. Also, any new line item on your NPDB record will often be reflexively reported to your medical board, who may then conduct their own investigation!

In conclusion

So far this book has been in service of the first goal we outlined in the introduction. I hope you now fully understand the peril you face should find yourself the focus of a complaint or disciplinary action. Now is not the time to be dismissive; the threat is real. This is an absolute threat to your professional wellbeing.

Protecting yourself and making it through this process, as mentioned, will require a lot of introspection and work. That is the focus of much of this book. However, you must survive long enough to be able to do that work. As such, the next chapter will focus first on immediate defensive actions.

CHAPTER THREE

Damage Control

Five things you should have already done

The moment your name is first mentioned in the same sentence as words like, "inappropriate," "disruptive," "poor communication," "boundaries," "peer review," or even just "complaint," you need to immediately realize that regardless of what happened or what you feel you did or did not do, your career is on the line.

As such, there are five things you need to immediately do and not do. Now many of these were touched upon already, but it is important to explicitly spell them out and list them as our starting point.

#1 - DO *treat this as seriously as you would a heart attack*

In our training, we were judged on our clinical acumen, technical skill, and patient outcomes. It was our sole job to get good at those things. Everything else was secondary.

As a result, it is common for this same mindset to persist once we are practicing on our own. If someone takes us to task on something we did, the first question we ask is, "How was the patient care?" Once we decide there was no issue there, we tend to want to move on.

The practical result of this is that we can be lackadaisical in our response to the types of complaints discussed in this book. This is absolutely the last thing you want to be. As stated, this is a real threat to your ability to practice.

As such, you need to promptly respond to any concerns raised regarding your speech or behavior. If someone requests a meeting, you must be proactive in making that happen as soon as possible. If someone asks you to review something and provide a response, you do it immediately and non-defensively. If you get an email about the issue at hand, you don't let in linger in your inbox waiting until you "get around to it."

In short, you need to be proactive and engaged. Others also need to perceive you as proactive and engaged. Anything less and it will be assumed that you do not care enough to take this issue seriously, which will not help you as the powers that be determine your future.

#2 - Do NOT *assume due process or transparency*

Remember administrative law and the two hard truths? If not, now is the time to go back and read the beginning of Chapter Two. Making these assumptions and forgetting the two hard truths is problematic for two reasons. First, it tends to make you passive early in the process. Second, it leaves you open to getting blindsided.

#3 - DO seek guidance early

Guidance can take many forms. A lawyer is a great form of guidance. Look for one who specializes in employment law - ideally one with experience with hospitals and medical boards. A senior peer or mentor can also be a great form of guidance. Especially someone who has been involved in these processes before and knows the ins and outs as well as the decision makers involved.

This book and the many resources online are also forms of guidance. You can find a lot out there, including advocacy groups for physicians facing similar challenges. But take everything with a grain of salt - this is the internet and everyone has an agenda.

The point is, this is not the time to go it alone. And yet, I am always surprised by how many physicians I work with say that they initially did consider speaking to an attorney or mentor, but then chose not to despite the fact that their ability to practice was at stake. I hear three consistent reasons as to why they made this decision.

First, they did not realize the gravity of the situation. They underestimated their institution's reaction to the situation and they failed to realize the power of the forces at play. Just as we discussed in Point #1 above, they assumed that because no poor patient outcome occurred, this type of complaint was less significant and would just "blow over."

Second, they were embarrassed. I get it. It's hard to reach out, to tell the story over and over and ask for help. But not as embarrassing or stressful as having a bad outcome from this process that potentially could have been mitigated.

Third, many physicians tell me that they did not seek counsel because they did not want to "escalate things" or make them "adversarial." I hope you now understand things have already escalated. Don't be fooled by the smiles and repetitive use of the word "voluntary."

At this point, having some form of counsel is generally going to be upside. For starters, in many of these types of administrative proceedings, you are allowed to have a lawyer or other advocate with you. They generally cannot argue for you or interject the way they would in a court of law, but they can observe and provide guidance. Also, they can interpret documentation (such as any complaint or your original contract) and help you draft effective responses. Finally, a lawyer can ensure that your rights are respected to the extent possible in this type of administrative process.

Having a lawyer is also a powerful signal. Physicians are incredibly risk and conflict-adverse . . . so are hospitals and medical boards. When you signal that you are engaged and willing to avail yourself of all resources, it may prompt a desire to resolve this by all parties more quickly. That may (and I emphasize *may*) give you a little leverage to come to a slightly better conclusion. Remember, at this point, a primary goal is to avoid an NPDB report or medical board sanction. It is also all about mitigating any wording used to describe the incident going forward (for example if a future employer calls your current hospital, what will the hospital say?).

#4 - Do NOT *voluntarily surrender privileges/licensure or quit in an effort to terminate proceedings*

The rationale for this was clearly laid out at the end of Chapter Two. It can be a huge mistake, and one that cannot be undone.

The truth is that until recently surrendering privileges while under investigation was a commonly used tactic to "get out of trouble." It made things easy for the hospital or medical board, as the problematic clinician was now gone. It often allowed the clinician to simply move to another organization or state, with no one the wiser. This was in fact partly why the NPDB was invented - to prevent this very scenario.

Now there may come a time when surrender of privileges / licensure or walking away is a rational choice. Just make sure that you absolutely understand the ramifications. Be very clear on NPDB reporting criteria. Perhaps even more important than that, make sure you understand what and to whom your hospital or medical board intends to report and what they will say if you take this option.

#5 - DO *shut up*

I know that sounds blunt, but I mean it. Stop talking. Stop interacting with people. Stop making small talk. Stop acting like your normal self.

The physician you were - that was yesterday. Today you are a clinical robot, at least for the immediate future. Come to work, do only what is essential for safe patient care that day, go home. No side conversations. No shop talk. No jokes. No social commentary. No opinion on anything unrelated to a clinical issue in front of you. No trying to improve "the system." No trying to teach other people through "constructive criticism." No discussing your weekend. No mention of the news. No opinions on other providers. No emotion. No friction. Someone consults you at 3am, you greet them with a smile and say "Thank you Sir, may I have another!"

Are you are starting to get the idea?

Now I realize this might sound extreme. I also realize it sounds untenable (and in the long run it is). But in the short run, it can be a career-saving move for three reasons:

First, whether or not you realize it, you are emotionally and cognitively compromised. In the immediate aftermath of being labeled a poor communicator, disruptive, or accused of a boundary violation, the stress is intense. Every time you go to work you are reminded of what is happening, and your stress response kicks in to overdrive. Your amygdala activates, which in turn inhibits your prefrontal cortex. As such, you are less able to engage in prefrontal functions such as perspective taking, emotional self-regulation, and nuanced decision making under stress.

Rather, you think more "limbically" - you are more reactive than responsive, you see mostly black and white, you repeat past behaviors that may be less useful in your current context. Neurocognitively, this is a terrible place to be when you are under the increased scrutiny of a PIP or workplace monitor. Limiting your behavioral repertoire as much as possible limits the risk of more problematic behavior until you can figure out what changes need to be made.

Second, everyone around you is now primed to misinterpret your behavior and look for problems. Two months ago, you could have made a comment or joke and it might not have been interpreted negatively. Now, you make the same comment or joke and others might be biased to interpret it in the most negative manner possible. Likewise, last week pushing back and advocating for a patient was just you being a good doctor. Today it is "disruptive behavior." Is this fair? Perhaps not. But it is the reality of having a target on your head. You don't want to give people even the smallest opportunity for misunderstanding or further friction.

Third, and perhaps most importantly, you may want to seriously limit your behavior because you may really be saying things that are offensive to others or doing things that make others uncomfortable.

We all have blind spots, some small, some large. Given what has happened to you, it is imperative that you assume that you may have some blind spot in your speech or your actions that has contributed to where you find yourself now.

Is it not at least *possible* that you:

- Are not fully aware of how your speech or behavior change under stress or when fatigued?

- Do not fully comprehend the power differential that you enjoy (due to privilege related to your title, age, gender, race, language, local culture, etc)
- Fail to see how your sense of humor or off-handed comments are coming at the expense of others
- Assume that, because you have other things in common, those around you must share your opinion / beliefs when in fact they do not
- Think that you are compartmentalizing other stressors in your life, when in fact they are impacting work.
- Spend more time being focused on being right or looking good, rather than being beneficial to others
- Are not aware of cultural differences that may create unintended friction
- Are lackadaisical about attention to non-clinical responsibilities and policies because they seem less important (ex: records compliance, your institution's electronics or data management policies, etc.)

Now I don't know if these or anything similar are true for you, but the point is *neither do you!* That is the definition of a blind spot.

It all comes down to Pascal's Wager

Essentially this is a version of Pascal's Wager. Either you have a blind spot that contributed to this situation, or you do not. One of those two things must be factually true. At the same time, there is no rational way for you to know which of those is true (definition of a blind spot - you can't see it).

Therefore you have two options going forward. One is to assume you may have a blind spot and significantly limit your speech and behavior until you have a chance to fully understand what that blind spot might be. The other option is to assume you don't have a blind spot, and change nothing.

If you do the former, and in fact have no blind spot, then you have inconvenienced yourself and made work less enjoyable in the short run. But if you do the latter, and do in fact have a blind spot, you may not be employed much longer. Which way are you going to err?

Maybe you figured this out already

Many physicians I work with have already taken this last step (Step #5). It is often a reflexive response. For many physicians, they have lived their career without any issues until this event. Now, suddenly they find themselves criticized and under scrutiny for what feels like "the consequences of just being themselves." At a loss as to how to proceed, many physicians just shut down and become a shell of their former selves. And it is difficult, as we can see in the example of Maha:

> *Maha was nephrologist in a large private group for the last 19 years. When she started it was a small, single hospital practice. Over time, her group bought out every competitor in the region. They also made some very savvy investments in dialysis centers. As such, the practice was extremely lucrative. At 20 years, every partner was allowed to retire with a seven-figure payout. But if they left sooner (or had a major negative administrative action), they got nothing.*
>
> *Unfortunately for Maha, she had had a couple of complaints in the last few years. Truth be told, she was a bit burned out. Also, she started doing a lot of work in a new hospital system her group acquired the contract for and it was a pretty toxic place. Until now these complaints were handled quietly by her practice head, but most recently a hospitalist reported her directly to HR and the CMO of the new hospital system. Her interactions were characterized as unprofessional and she found herself under a zero-*

tolerance contract that her group agreed to in order to appease the new CMO.

By the time I began working with her, she had shut down completely. She previously considered herself personable, talkative, and enjoyed the social aspect of work. Now she just punched the clock, never complaining or saying anything to anyone. She was, by her own admission, clearly miserable. But when I tried to work with her and see if there wasn't some way she could be more of herself, she replied with, "Its just too risky, I could lose 1.4 million dollars."

Every coaching session with Maha came back to this same sticking point. Despite my attempts to help her create new strategies or skills, Maha stuck with her plan. People kept asking her at work, "Whats wrong?" or, "Are you ok?" But she did not care. She kept her head down, her mouth closed, and 7 months later to the day she hit the 20 year mark and immediately put in her notice.

Now she is on a beach somewhere.

Maha's story is informative for two reasons. First, it shows how challenging it can be to shut down and not be yourself. Although I think it is important to do so in the immediate aftermath of this situation, it must be acknowledged that it is a big ask that adds more stress onto an already stressful situation. It is not workable long term.

Second, it does show that in *some* unique situations, maybe it is the only strategy you need. If you are leaving clinical medicine permanently in the next 6 months, it may not be worth doing the hard work and introspection that the rest of this book will entail.

But most of us are not in Maha's unique situation. Most of us have years of clinical practice that we are looking forward to. As such, shutting down forever is not a viable strategy. It will burn us out and bring our career to a premature end, just in a different way. What most of us need is a way to discover our blind spots, a way to change elements in our work and our lives to improve the quality of our days, and a way to develop new skills so that we will not ever harm others through our speech or behavior again.

That brings us to our third goal and the focus of the remainder of this book. Each of the chapters that follows takes a focused look at one area of our lives or one particular skill set. Although the chapters could be approached in an a la carte fashion, I highly recommend you read all of them and in order. If you think a chapter is particularly not applicable to you, I challenge you that perhaps it may be the most important one for you to read (remember blind spots?).

CHAPTER FOUR

Blind Spots

The stories that we tell ourselves

As an executive coach, I spend my days talking to high-performing professionals. I listen to their stories about themselves and about the world. I can tell you with certainty that even the most high-functioning of us engage in a little self-serving bias here and there as we create narratives about our own lives. Most often, this is because our brains are hard-wired to avoid distress, and so we often create narratives motivated more by our own emotional and cognitive comfort rather than a complete and clear assessment of reality. And if you think you this does not apply to you, I can prove that it does right now.

If you are reading this as a physician, you are in the top 1% of educated people in the world. You are in the top 1% of income earners in the world. You have a title, "doctor," that earns you immediate social status in any situation. You work in a profession idolized on TV and in movies. By just about any criteria, you are extremely successful. So, I ask you, how have you accomplished this? In other words, what is the story that you tell yourself (and maybe others) of your success?

Is it one of incredible hard work and perseverance? Does your narrative include thoughts about how you delayed gratification and sacrificed, when others lacked self-control? Do you reflect upon your ability to cultivate vision, passion, or perhaps even a sense of calling to get through those low moments? Maybe you attribute your ability to rise up to challenge after challenge to your grit, which you honed through years of applying yourself and always taking the hard road?

Take a moment before reading on, and really reflect upon your narrative regarding your success as a professional . . .

Now I want to challenge you.

In your narrative, how much do you acknowledge the role that luck has played in your life? Does your story talk about how lucky you are to have had no physical or mental health problems that would have made pursuing a path in medicine impossible? What about the luck of where, when, or to what family you were born?

Do you reflect on those moments of pure serendipity? The chance event that had a major influence on your path? The unexpected person who played a major role or who presented you with a critical opportunity?

What about those times you just happened to guess right on a test, and those few extra points subsequently made all the difference in a grade or class rank? What about the fact that there was that one person on the admissions committee who pushed just a little bit harder for you because of some obscure and irrelevant background element in your application that resonated with them, when otherwise there was nothing to differentiate you from the other 1000 amazing applicants?

Or how about genetics? The research is overwhelming that intelligence is almost entirely genetic. Your ability to focus for extraordinary lengths of time, your ability to memorize vast volumes of information, your ability to think deeply and critically - these are nothing more than the result of a lucky role of the genetic dice.

Yet most of us dramatically under-emphasize the role that these elements have played in our success. To really recognize them would be to acknowledge that things aren't nearly as in our control as we like to believe. It would be saying that we perhaps deserve less credit for what we have accomplished, and that thought is simply too emotionally and cognitively uncomfortable. We've worked too hard.

Likewise, people who perceive themselves as unsuccessful dramatically *overestimate* the influence that luck, genetics, and serendipity have had on their struggle - because similarly that is the more comfortable version of events for them - "I just never got a lucky break," or "the deck was stacked against me, there was nothing I could do."

Regardless, the point is this: It is human nature to prioritize emotional and cognitive comfort over accuracy and completeness in the narratives we tell ourselves about our lives and the events of the world around us.

So with that in mind, it is now time to ask you the million dollar question:

What might you be ignoring about the events that have led you to read this book?

If you are reading this book because of an administrative review or disciplinary process, you likely have a narrative as to what happened regarding that process. You have a story as to who did what, how things came to be, your culpability or lack thereof, others' motives, etc. It is likely that this narrative prioritizes cognitive and emotional comfort *at least somewhere* within it, thus obscuring a complete and objective analysis of events. When we are caught up in these incomplete or skewed stories, "hooked" by them so to speak, it is almost impossible to make meaningful change. We must explore them and challenge them if we are to move forward.

While only you can identify your own narratives, there are a few common themes that I see in my work. The following are offered as examples of how powerful narratives can be and how we can get stuck. Four examples for your consideration are:

- The "Where is the grit?" story
- The "I was advocating for the patient" story
- The "They are out to get me" story
- The "They didn't get X right, therefore this whole thing is BS" story

The "Where is the grit?" story

Do you find yourself lamenting that people are just too sensitive these days? Does it seem like those around you lack work ethic? Does no one have any backbone? If these thoughts feel familiar, the "Where is the grit?" story may be a part of your narrative.

Generally, this narrative goes something like this:

> *Younger generations have been too coddled. They were raised by helicopter parents who shielded them from all adversity. Everyone was given a trophy, even when they did terribly. Now those younger generations are percolating through the medical ranks as physicians, nurses, etc. The result is that no one is wiling to work hard. They cannot handle adversity and "push through" when needed. They settle for mediocrity, and can't handle criticism of any kind. They prioritize themselves over their patients. They cannot engage in intellectual debate because they are too fragile and easily offended . . .*

These are not uncommon thoughts and feelings for the clinicians I work with. Many of these same clinicians feel that this is the reason that they themselves were labeled problematic. It's not that their own speech or behavior was actually *unacceptable*; rather, the problem is really that everyone around them is too *unaccepting* of any semblance of discomfort.

The problem with these thoughts, however, is that for every behavior that you may believe demonstrates a lack of grit, there is a counter-argument that others will make that the same behavior is a character strength.

For example, perhaps when you were a resident your attendings were brutal. High expectations, 36 hour work days, and being thrashed for every little mistake were the norm. That adversity was the forge that molded you into an exceptional physician - and its a travesty that those that are following behind you can't hack it.

Or is it? Older generations of physicians have the highest burnout rate of any educated professional. They also have the highest suicide rate, the highest life dissatisfaction, and the lowest number of close friends / strong social connections. Ninety percent of physicians would not recommend their career to their own child. Seeing this, medical students lament that they cannot find mentors whose professional or personal lives that they want to emulate. So is the rejection of traditional medical culture by younger generations really a sign of weakness, or is it a rational response to the toxicity that they are observing? Is it an attempt to re-shape the culture of medicine into something workable going forward?

Consider another thought - that everyone is more easily offended and too sensitive, whether this be in response to a joke or as part of an intellectual debate. Is this a lack of grit, or a function of the radically different world that they were raised in? The content that they have encountered online since childhood is more extreme and upsetting than ever before - unchecked racist diatribes, extreme porn, sexist trolling - just to name a few. Is it really a surprise that given what they have been bombarded with, younger generations are more concerned with having boundaries and demanding civility? Is it surprising they focus more on impact, and less on intent because they have far more experience seeing how speech and action harm others in often insidious ways?

Now I present these points and counterpoints not to try to convince you that you are wrong. Rather, I am simply demonstrating that what you label a lack of grit may well be labeled by others as positive. Most importantly, it is critical to realize that as an individual, **you are not the final arbiter of what is acceptable** or unacceptable in terms of behavior, commitment, communication, and boundaries in medicine. *Society is.* And what is acceptable at a societal level has shifted dramatically in recent years.

Now your behaviors, communication style, and expectations of others may have been completely rational, *and perhaps necessary*, for surviving your formative professional years. That does not, however, make them inherently right or better. The problem lies in when you take behaviors and expectations that worked in one context (your training), and carry them forward blindly into a new context (the current healthcare landscape). In a nutshell, this is how many physicians run into trouble - the context and societal expectations have changed, but their behaviors have not.

Constantly viewing those around you as lacking, and lamenting that they do not share the same professional development and worldview, is exhausting for you and stressful for them. So if you find yourself hooked by the "Where's the grit" story, you will likely have to change your expectations around behavior, communication, and expectations of others if you wish to continue to practice. In particular, the upcoming chapters on civility and communications may be particularly helpful.

The "I was advocating for the patient" story

It used to be that all transgressions would be forgiven if they were committed "for the good of the patient." Yelling at nurses, throwing scalpels, tearing apart a resident for an oversight - all overlooked in the name of education and patient safety.

Not anymore. Now you are expected to keep the patient safe while also promoting psychological safety for those around you. It is expected that while navigating the incredible stressors of day to day practice, you also listen well, promote respect, lead by example, and cultivate a growth mindset for those around you.

This is a tall order, and again, the challenge relates to how we developed as professionals. In our training, we learned early on to internalize the patient's well-being. In a very paternalistic way, we were taught to medically and legally accept 100% responsibility for that person's life. When a resident missed an important lab, or when a colleague moved too slowly, we learned to react as if we were being directly threatened, and that kind of internalization has its benefits in medicine where lives are literally at stake. At the same time, it also results in our stress response being repeatedly activated at a very high level - which negatively shapes our behavior.

Now you may recall from medical school the neuroanatomy of the stress response. When stressed, our amygdala and other limbic structures activate. They inhibit our prefrontal cortex and we have reduced executive function. For example, we are less able to see nuances, less able to take others' perspectives, and, perhaps most importantly, we lose emotional down-regulation. Instead of thinking and responding with our best selves, we become more reactive and engage in limbic thinking.

Some neuroscientists like to call this the "reptilian brain." Evolutionarily a much older part of our brain, deep brain structures like the amygdala engage in "fight or flight" type responses. We see things as black and white. We approach everything with a negative bias. We regress to old behaviors despite new contexts. This was evolutionarily very useful for surviving tiger attacks, but it is problematic for dealing with the nuances of modern life.

At a practical level, this usually manifests as uncivil behavior - raising your voice, using aggressive body language to get your point across, trying to be right, criticizing or belittling others, etc. Again, 15 years ago these behaviors were not only tolerated but expected. Today they will cost you your ability to practice. And here lies the rub - our medical and legal responsibility has not lessened, and our brains have not evolved in how they respond to stress, and we are expected to be *responsive* despite our brain being hardwired to be *reactive*.

We are increasingly held to a higher standard of civility despite an increasingly stressful practice environment with brains that still think we are being chased by tigers. We can no longer justify our own reactive incivility in the name of patient safety. So if the "I was advocating for the patient" story rings true for you, you may be particularly interested in the skillset to be discussed in the next chapter (The Civil War).

The "They are out to get me" story

Do you believe that what has happened is nothing more than a ruse to get rid of you? Sure, you said or did something that was not in accord with your best self, but the powers that be are blowing it out of proportion. Everyone else gets away with the same behaviors, but they are targeting you and using it as an excuse to make life uncomfortable in an attempt to force you out. If this rings true, you likely have the "They are out to get me" story as part of your narrative.

This narrative is particularly powerful. Instead of engaging with the idea that your behavior was not acceptable, this narrative allows you to dismiss your behavior as "not the real problem." Rather, the "real problem" is other people who are weaponizing this event.

There is just one problem with this narrative - they don't need a ruse to get rid of you, so why in the world would they engage in this convoluted and time-intensive process?

First of all, if you are an employed physician (which greater than 50% of us now are), I can virtually promise you that in your contract there is a "Termination Without Cause" clause. Read it and you will discover that in most cases you can be let go any time, without a reason being given, with very little notice (usually 30 days).

Now if you are in a private practice group, it may be a little more difficult. However, even most groups have a process for letting a partner go without cause, and the requirements for that are often less stringent than you might think. If they want you gone, it will happen.

Lastly, if you have hospital privileges those too can often be revoked at any time, again without cause and with very little notice. If you don't believe me, I encourage you to read the fine print of your privileges contract. You will likely be very surprised at how little protection and recourse you have.

All of this, by the way, also assumes that they do not have cause. Poor communication, incivility, boundary violations, disruptive behavior - these are all fair game for terminating you or your privileges *for cause* and are likely also stipulated in your contract. Again, referring to Chapter Two, the threshold for such accusations being founded is low. Innocence is not presumed. The standard is not the high bar of "beyond a reasonable doubt." Chances are, given the way that most contracts are written, they already have more than enough to let you go with *or* without cause.

So the point is this - it is already easy to get rid of you. So why would an organization go through the incredible machinations of PIPs, PHP referrals, and the like? After all, it is a lot of work on their part. Meetings, phone calls, suspensions, referrals, paperwork, workplace monitors, more meetings, more emails, etc. It also often opens the organization up to more liability than simply just firing you. So again, why do it?

The reason why, and you may not believe this, is that they *don't* want to let you go. This is usually for one of two reasons. One, they sincerely want to keep you but your behavior or speech isn't in accord with the organization's standards. They need things to improve, and to protect themselves legally they need to be proactive in making this happen. Or two, they simply can't afford to let go of you right now, because you bring in too much revenue or are too hard to replace.

In either case, there is an opportunity for you to make meaningful changes and find a way forward that is workable for the organization and for you, but only if you are willing to entertain the possibility that there is something to their criticisms of your behavior.

The "They didn't get X right, therefore this whole thing is BS" story

At this point in your journey, you have likely told your version of events many times to many people. In turn, they have synthesized this information along with other data and created their own story of events, which they in turn have shared with others. It is like the old childhood game of telephone where one person whispers something to someone, who in turn whispers what they thought they heard to a third person, and so one down the line until the end where it is hilariously distorted.

Similarly, there is likely some distortion somewhere in the accounting of events to this point. Perhaps your referral letter to the PHP said there were four problematic incidents, but your Chief of Staff swears there were only three. Maybe in your third-party assessment they reversed where you went to college and medical school.

When these inevitable factual errors occur, it can be tempting to seize upon them as proof of incompetence. We are, after all, nothing if not perfectionists. If they can't even get the small stuff right, how can they be trusted to understand the big picture? We can get wrapped up in small errors and inconsistencies and use them to reassure ourselves that therefore nothing about this process is correct or valid.

> *Monty was an interventional radiologist in a medium-sized urban hospital. Over the last few years there had been multiple incidents of incivility - mostly being passive-aggressive or condescending to non-physician staff. Given how much revenue he brought in, these incidents were often overlooked. Recently, however, a new CMO had been appointed who was less willing to ignore these behaviors. The result was an escalating process of verbal warnings, written warnings, and ultimately a suspension with a PHP referral.*
>
> *In my first conversation with Monty, before I could even say a word, he immediately launched into, "Let me tell you what's really going on . . . " He then spoke at length about how he and the Chief of Staff never got along (they trained at the same program), and that that Chief had it out for him for years. Furthermore, the Chief of Staff and the new CMO were golf buddies, and so clearly both were together against him. After all, no one else got in trouble for acting the exact same way! Also, the most recent incident involved a medical student who initiated a conversation on a controversial topic, and Monty was convinced that the medical student was asked by the Chief of Staff to set him up.*

As further proof, Monty walked me through both his organization's and the PHP's evaluations. First, he was adamant that their similarity meant that they were in cahoots. He then proceeded to point out small errors line by line. One report said he came dressed in "a blazer, slacks, a dress shirt, and a tie." Monty was apoplectic, because he had worn a matching suit! Another document said he was born in Utah, but actually he was born in Nevada and moved to Utah when he was two years old. Referring to one of the older incidents of concern, the synopsis noted he got into a verbal altercation with another attending over a consult - but it was a fellow, not an attending! And they got the campus wrong, it happened at one of the satellite facilities! This was all proof of incompetence by everyone involved. Furthermore, it showed that the PHP was really not interested in his version of events, but was just doing his organization's bidding.

Both the "They are out to get me," and the "They didn't get X right, therefore this whole thing is BS" narratives were very strong for Monty. Whenever we tried to focus on creating goals around behavior or exploring what interpersonal skills might be of use in the future, he would often get hooked by one of these narratives, which made progress very, very hard.

What are your narratives?

I present these four narratives as food for thought. For most physicians I work with, at least one narrative will resonate with them.

Only you can identify and explore your own narratives about the events that have transpired. A powerful process for doing this is the "My Narrative" Exercise that can be found in Appendix One. Before reading further, I strongly encourage you to use this tool to explore your own narratives and challenge them, so that you can make the most use of the chapters that follow.

CHAPTER FIVE

The Civil War

Incivility in all of its guises

Having explored your narrative and its potential blind spots, it is now time to get more granular and focus on the specific behaviors that often lead to disciplinary action. For so many physicians that I have worked with, the behaviors that they are being called to task on revolve around one word - *incivility* - and so that is as good a place as any to start to see if this applies to your situation.

Incivility is a slippery concept. We know it when we see it in others, but it is much harder to objectively define. It is even harder to see it in ourselves. In an effort to understand this concept, it is best to start by examining where incivility fits on the spectrum of physician behavior.

PROFESSIONAL BEHAVIOR		UNPROFESSIONAL BEHAVIOR	
Healthy	Incivility ⟶	Unethical conduct ⟶	Criminal
		Propagating medical misinformation	
	Interrupting others		
Strong communication			Falsifying billing
		Threatening to get others in trouble	
Appropriate boundaries	Belittling		Hiding mistakes
	Ignoring requests for help		
		Financial kickbacks	
Beneficence	Yelling		Ignoring consent
		Dual relationships	
	Rolling your eyes		Diverting narcotics

Diagram 1 - The Professional / Unprofessional Spectrum

Starting at the far right end of the spectrum, we have actions that are so unprofessional that they are illegal. These are codified into administrative or criminal law, and include things like physically assaulting a patient, billing fraud, and diverting narcotics. We know exactly what these things are, because we can look at federal or state statutes that tell us exactly what we can't do. These things are black and white.

Moving back along the spectrum of unprofessional behavior, next we have unethical behavior. While not illegal, these are still highly problematic behaviors that are not acceptable within our profession. For example, dual relationships (where you are treating someone with whom you also have a sexual relationship or a significant financial relationship) are unethical. Another example would be promoting medical ideas or treatments that are not evidence-based or keeping with the standard of care, especially for secondary gain like fame or money. While there are guidelines and policies around many of these things, it is impossible to anticipate all unethical behavior. Therefore what is unethical is generally determined by our peers through mechanisms such as medical boards or medical executive committees.

Last, even further left on the spectrum we come to incivility. Incivility is a subset of unprofessional behavior characterized by less intense actions that are nonetheless harmful to patients or colleagues, although often in indirect and subtle ways that are more cumulative in their effect ("death by a thousand paper cuts"). Common examples in healthcare include:

Verbal incivility:

- Belittling or putting others down
- Speaking ill of or gossiping about colleagues / other departments / the institution
- Interrupting others
- Criticizing others in front of colleagues or patients
- Yelling or raising your voice
- Playing favorites

- Taking credit for others' good work while placing blame on others for mistakes
- Threatening to write someone up or get them in trouble
- Charting in a derogatory manner regarding other providers, patients, or their families

Somatic incivility (using the body and other non-verbal cues)

- Violating other's personal space, especially during heated communications
- Throwing your hands in the air, slamming a fist on the table, throwing objects in frustration
- Rolling your eyes or refusing to make eye contact
- Turning your back on someone mid-interaction

Incivility through opting out / inaction

- Ignoring consults or requests for help
- Refusing to document conversations or write a note when requested
- Disappearing when a problem arises or is anticipated
- Being significantly behind on documentation or orders, impacting other's work flow

Incivility is often in the eye of the beholder, i.e. the recipient of the speech or behavior. Just as we stated in Chapter Two, if someone feels you were condescending, aggressive in your body language, inappropriate with a joke, blowing them off, etc., you will have a hard time convincing them or others otherwise. In that sense, it is the least well-defined of the three categories of unprofessional behavior.

Finally, everything on the professional-unprofessional spectrum is also slowly moving to the right. Things that were considered uncivil a few years ago are now also explicitly unethical according to our state medical board position statements. Behavior that may have been normalized during our training as "just how medicine works" is now recognized for the incivility it really is. Incivility is therefore a dynamic concept at the edge of the professional and the unprofessional.

The control agenda

Given this, how are we to know incivility? We tend to know it when we see it in others, so there must be some instinctive litmus test we are using. Yet it is so hard to see in ourselves, so can we develop that litmus test for our own behavior?

At its core, uncivil behavior is an attempt to *control* distress or dissatisfaction. This is uniquely different from the other types of unprofessional behavior discussed. Illegal and unethical behaviors are almost always motivated by personal gain, psychopathology, or large lapses in judgement. By contrast, incivility is almost always motivated by the agenda of emotional control. When we are experiencing distress or dissatisfaction in the form of difficult thoughts, feelings, or memories related to the work in front of us, we want to exert control and make those thoughts and feelings go away.

This is best demonstrated through examples. Let's look first at some common examples of difficult thoughts, feelings, and memories that many physicians may find familiar:

- "I cant believe that nurse is on again, she calls me more than all of the other nurses on that floor combined. Guess I'm not sleeping tonight!"
- "Why are they asking me to consult again? They didn't bother implementing my recommendations two days ago. Of course the patient is worse and they expect me to magically fix it?
- "That patient came to the ER for what? A bug bite? Literally?"
- "This is the exact same scenario I got sued for four years ago."

And of course how do we respond to these uncomfortable thoughts? With incivility of course! When the nurse calls, we passive-aggressively make him or her feel stupid in the hopes that they will think twice about calling again. When a team doesn't implement our recommendations the first time, we drag our feet and let them know they are a low priority on the second consult. When we do get around to the consult we don't hesitate to to say I told you so and launch into a condescending lecture. Or in the third case above, we go in the ER room with the patient with the bug bite and we don't make eye contact, spend all of 20 seconds on the exam, and discharge them before they are even registered. Last, when we see a case that was a disaster for us previously, we dodge it in the hopes it will fall to another colleague.

Being condescending, confrontational, physically aggressive, opting out, looking good, being right, getting our needs met, demanding perfection — in the immediate moment these all feel *so good* because it feels like we are doing something to get rid of the source of our discomfort.

To some extent this works, at least in the short run. The nurse often does shrink away. We do get to lecture the providers requesting the consult. The patient goes to a different ER next time. We dodge the case that scares us. This satiates our stress response because we have done something about the "threat." In turn, the behavior is thus self-reinforcing even though it may be unworkable in the long run.

The opposite of control

If we weren't motivated by control, if we could instead hold these difficult thoughts and feelings more lightly and pivot to our best selves, what would our motivation be then? We would be motivated by a desire to solve the problem in a way that serves the other party involved. We would engage respectfully and constructively. Others would trust our intent as holding goodwill for them. In other words, we would be motivated by *beneficence.*

This is the litmus test. In a given interaction, are we *reactive* and motivated by emotional control for ourselves, or are we *responsive* and motivated by beneficence for the other? If the former, there is a good chance incivility may manifest. The other party may not always register it, and we may not always get in trouble for it, but it is always potentially there when our focus is avoiding or eliminating difficult thoughts and feelings.

So how do we cultivate the ability to see this in ourselves in real time and embrace beneficence? It is one thing to talk about it, and it is another to use this idea to improve our experience of our work. To this end, there are a few tools I use with the physicians I work with.

First, I will often ask them to spend a few days simply looking for incivility in others and writing down what they see and hear. This is often eye opening. Incivility in medicine is epidemic. All too often, we just don't see it because it has been normalized. Usually within a few days my clients have pages of examples, and are already starting to see where they might be doing the same to others.

Next, I have them practice using the Control Spectrum Worksheet found in Appendix Two. Usually I will ask them to fill it out once a day for about 2 weeks. First, I have them think of a challenging interaction or a moment of poor behavior on their part. If you wish, you can do this right now using an event or interaction that prompted you to read this book. In one to two succinct sentences, factually write down the situation. Then, again in 1-2 sentences, you write down how you reacted to the situation. Make sure you think about verbal and non-verbal behavior (and remember opting out / inaction is a behavior).

Now, being completely honest with yourself, where would you put yourself on the spectrum of control versus beneficence as your motivation in that moment? Control is about controlling the uncomfortable thoughts, feelings, and memories that come up in the situation. Control can thus take many forms:

- Behavior to get rid of unwanted people or events (ex: yelling at a nurse so they think twice about calling in the future)
- Getting our immediate needs met such as what you feel you deserve (ex: demanding respect)
- Looking good / Being right
- Feeling powerful or in control
- Getting rid of pressure
- Motivating self or others through coercion, embarrassment, or threat

Keeping these in mind, use a pen to mark where you were on the line. If you acted completely out of an agenda of control, put the X all the way to the left, if you acted solely out of beneficence, put the X all the way to the right (honesty is key here, no one will see this but you). The truth is often there are elements of both, so you can put the X anywhere along the line that feels correct. Now spend a few moments answering the subsequent questions on the worksheet.

The power of this exercise is that it builds self awareness. Although you are doing this in hindsight, every time you do it you are reinforcing neural pathways that eventually will allow you to do it in the heat of the moment. Whether you call this self-awareness, cognitive flexibility, or mindfulness, it is perhaps the most important tool we can develop as physicians. It is the ability to pause in challenging moments, see what is happening more objectively, and pivot to our best selves. It is the difference between being reactive versus being responsive. Developing this skill will go a long way in avoiding further behaviors others might consider problematic.

However, this is a skill that must be practiced. It is like learning the guitar. You can read about how to play a guitar, and listen to lectures about guitar technique, but at the end of the day you will only improve if you *play* the guitar. The skillset we have just discussed is similar. So if you find yourself wanting more practice, there are many resources out there. Mindfulness Based Stress Reduction courses (MBSR) have been used to great effect to build this skillset specifically in physicians. There are also compassion-based cognitive training courses for healthcare providers that cover many of the same ideas. Working with a coach is a more tailored, focused way to build this skill. It also creates a structure for ongoing accountability. If self-study is more your thing, I strongly recommend looking into Acceptance and Commitment Therapy (ACT). There are great resources online as well as books, in particular those by Russ Harris.

CHAPTER SIX

Off Limits!

A dozen things you just shouldn't
talk about at work

Incivility often plays a role in why many physicians find themselves under administrative review. Sometimes it goes by another name, like "disruptive behavior," or "poor communication." Regardless, we have all done it. Thus, examining our own tendencies towards incivility is an important first step.

Incivility is not the only way we can violate someone's boundaries, however. We can cause harm by talking about inappropriate topics, by giving unwanted opinions, or by failing to recognize our privilege as it relates to certain topics. These can easily occur even though our intent was well-meaning.

More simply stated, sometimes we just put our foot in our mouth. Say something stupid. Phrase something in a way that is offensive. Engage in conversation we have no business engaging in. Sometimes we fail to recognize others' perspectives and lived experiences. Thus it is not enough just to avoid incivility; rather, we must also be mindful of the pitfalls of everyday conversation even when we think we are being well-meaning. To avoid these pitfalls, we must first understand the factors that make it so easy to communicate poorly.

Human communication is a set-up for misunderstanding

Countless neuroscience studies have shown that when we engage in communication, we bring our own thinking biases to the conversation. We see what is said through the lens of our worldview and personal privilege, our past experiences, and our current emotional state. All of these in turn inform our interpretation of what was just said.

Think back to the narrative exercise you did in Chapter 4 ("Blind spots"). When you wrote your story, what percentage of it was your interpretation of events versus indisputable fact? Likely most of it. The same phenomenon occurs every moment of every conversation. This is why two people can walk away from a seemingly straightforward conversation with two completely different interpretations of what was said and what was intended.

Its hard to stop "doctoring"

As if communication was not hard enough, our tendencies as physicians make it even worse. We are particularly prone to poor conversational boundaries because of our professional identity. After all, at work we are paid to solve problems and give our opinion, often very quickly. We are constantly required to think critically and play devil's advocate. We are the team leader who others often defer to for final decision making.

Given this role of "expert" that we constantly play, it's not surprising that we have a hard time switching this off. We often have very strong opinions about everything (not just medicine) and we like to share those, too. We have a tendency to jump in and try to problem solve everything. We may also assume that our opinion holds more weight regardless of the topic. Adding insult to injury, most of those around us have no choice but to listen to us when we do engage them because of the hierarchy of medicine.

Thus *we* may feel that we are engaging in healthy, intellectual conversation by debating both sides of an issue, but the other person may see us as refusing to denounce a harmful position. Another person may just want to be listened to and emotionally validated, but we pepper them with "helpful" solutions to a situation we have no first hand perspective on. We may think another person is interested in engaging with us, when in reality they just don't know how to get out of an unwanted conversation or they feel they can't openly disagree with us due to medical hierarchy.

Hot-button topics make everything worse

Misunderstandings happen under the best of circumstances. As we just saw, our "doctoring" habits don't help either. Add to this an emotional or controversial topic and you have the trifecta of communication disasters.

Consider the research of neuroscientists Liane Young and Rebecca Saxe. They have consistently demonstrated that when people engage in a conversation regarding topics that are more emotional or taboo (such as sex, politics, or race), that people are far more likely to ignore the intent behind what is said and focus far more on the impact. The more controversial the topic, the more intent is disregarded, even when engaging with people we may know well.

Thus for all of the above reasons, there are simply topics of conversation that should be avoided in most work settings. Easily 95% of incidents of poor communication and verbal boundary violations are the result of venturing into one of the twelve topics that follow.

But before I go through these I must make an important caveat. I am not saying that these topics are to *never* be discussed in the workplace. It has been shown that discussing challenging topics, such as race or gender, can actually improve psychological safety in the workplace which in turn improves professional relationships and performance. However, this must be done in a very specific way to be beneficial. It must be intentional - pre-planned with all parties consenting to engage. There need to be clearly defined goals for the conversation. It should be done in a neutral, safe space. There should be ground rules for the discussion, and ideally, a moderator as well.

In other words, what I am saying is that these 12 topics are not "water cooler" talk. They should not be brought up casually, or in the spirit of intellectual debate to pass the time in the doctor's lounge or OR.

1. Sex and intimate relationships

Sex and intimacy are natural parts of human existence but they have no place being discussed at work.

Surveys consistently show that people feel that sexuality is the number one most inappropriate topic for the workplace, even more than religion or politics. While you may feel comfortable discussing these aspects of yourself, many people will not appreciate hearing about them. And they absolutely don't want to hear what you have to say about *their* sex life or sexuality.

Furthermore, if someone feels that you have created an offensive work environment with your commentary, they may have grounds to claim sexual harassment. A sexual harassment claim is just about the most damaging form of complaint that can be made against you, and can be crippling for moving forward and continuing to work.

2. Money and income

Chances are you make more, *a lot more*, than the people you work with. Talking about income and spending can easily lead to jealousy in those you work with every day. This in turn can reduce their work performance and satisfaction, which is going to impact you.

Furthermore, studies have shown that people who constantly talk about money at work are perceived as less competent and less dedicated. Simple comments, such as how a patient or procedure is worth so many RVUs, can be interpreted as being in it "only for the money." Likewise, when you are complaining about someone's performance or systemic issues it can undermine your argument if you phrase things in terms of negatively impacting reimbursement or bonuses (rather than patient safety).

3. Religion and spirituality

We all have religious and spiritual beliefs, even if those beliefs are to have no beliefs. Chances are we feel very strongly about those. So does everyone else. In other words, religious and spiritual beliefs tend to have a major impact on our world view and perhaps even our choice of vocation, and they may differ greatly from those of the person standing next to us.

As such, they are the epitome of hot button topics that neurocognitively impair our ability to perspective take, think abstractly, and down-regulate strong emotions. No wonder this is one of two things you should never discuss at Thanksgiving dinner!

4. Politics

People often have very strongly held views on politics. Unlike religion, we often engage in political conversations with the goal of persuasion and debate. The potential for such conversations going awry is very, very high - particularly in today's political climate.

Also, such conversations are unlikely to be of any benefit. The types of "healthy debate" that occur in the workplace around politics are more likely to entrench others' views and cause them to bristle. Are you really engaging in such conversations for the beneficence of others? Is there mostly only downside to these conversations? Absolutely.

5. Bodies and physical abilities

It should go without saying that we should not make comments about peoples' appearance, weight, bodies, or physical abilities in our day-to-day lives. Yet it is also important to note that this contrasts directly with our work, where all we do is talk about peoples' bodies and physical abilities. To us, bodies are not people. Rather, they are meat puzzles we need to solve. As such, we can be inadvertently cavalier and callous when talking about others' bodies and abilities. Likewise we can forget that our carte blanche to discuss bodies only applies to our patients (and even then there are limits).

While most of us still manage to avoid saying overtly *negative* things about someone's body or abilities, we often don't hesitate to make "helpful" observations or positive statements, especially if they relate to health. Unfortunately, these are often not wanted or can be received in a way other than intended. Pointing out how it's great that a person lost weight, or that their botox looks good, or how well they compensate for an injury or disability may all *seem* complimentary. However, it may not be appreciated by the receiver. Maybe they don't want this discussed in front of others, even if they brought it up themselves at another time!

It is critical to remember that the majority of physicians who get in trouble in regards to comments about others' bodies actually get in trouble for seemingly neutral or positive comments. People just don't want their bodies and abilities discussed at work, and certainly not by a physician who is not their physician.

6. Race and ethnicity

Having difficult conversations about race at work is necessary for an equitable and inclusive workplace. Similarly, having difficult conversations about racism in medicine is critical for eliminating healthcare disparities. As stated above, however, these are conversations that should be intentional. They need to be planned and held in a structured way with all parties in agreement as to the purpose and goals.

Problems tend to occur when these topics are brought up casually. When they appear in our day-to-day conversation or in the context of current events there is more opportunity for misunderstanding or negating another's lived experience. It's important to remember that everyone's personal experience is different - even among two people who identify as having the same race or ethnicity. Therefore, talking about the personal impact of race or ethnicity, debating what constitutes a race or ethnicity, or comparing and contrasting one's experiences, are all fraught with the possibility of inadvertently coming across as adversarial or racist.

7. Gender and sexuality

Gender and sexual orientation are at the core of our being, and thus highly personal. For all the same reasons cited above, engaging in meaningful conversations around this topic in the day-to-day workplace is unnessecary.

Also, this is another situation in which we need to be careful to not "doctor." As medically trained scientists, there is actually a lot we can say about the science of gender. We know a lot about the biology and genetics of what it means to be part of a species that sexually reproduces. When we put our doctor hat on, however, we run the risk of "empiricizing" another's emotional, lived experience.

8. Jokes and humor

Humor is a wonderful thing, and it is often used as a tool for dealing with the stressors of our sometimes dark profession. The challenge with humor, however, is that it almost always comes at the expense of someone.

Think of the funniest moments or jokes you've experienced lately. How many of those did not involve some item on this list? Not many. In fact, things usually aren't really funny unless they are witty or edgy or embarrassing for someone. Hence why jokes like "Why did the chicken cross the road?" just don't cut it anymore for us as adults. It's not that humor can never be used, but you need to be extremely careful as to who that humor might be at the expense of.

9. Family matters

Like sexuality and imitate relationships, people do not want to hear about your family relationships or drama at work. Beyond the basic, "What did you do with your kids this weekend?" or, "How is your partner?" no one really wants you to spill the tea.

Fair or not, it's also important to remember that people judge your competency in the workplace by your overall perceived competence in every area of your life. When you reveal friction occurring in other areas of your life, especially if you complain, get personal, or blame others, you are judged negatively regarding your professional skillset.

One exception worth noting, however, is that if you have had a major life event that might impact your performance. A divorce or a death are going to be virtually impossible to compartmentalize and will impact your workday. In this instance, you may want to tell your supervisor or close colleagues. If you do so, you should divulge basic, factual details and focus on how this might impact work - do not get into personal details.

10. Health problems

You would think that of all people who could understand health challenges, it would be our colleagues in medicine. Unfortunately, the same rules apply as just mentioned under "Family matters." Health issues are perceived as weakness and professional incompetence. Even our "work friends" are likely only to care about how your health issue may impact them (their call schedule, patient load, etc) and hold it against you. It is absolutely not fair, but it is true.

Just as above, however, if a health issue is going to have a major impact on work, there may be a scenario in which you should share limited factual information as it pertains to work performance. If you find yourself in a scenario of this magnitude your first step should actually be to speak with an attorney to understand your medical rights. Ironically, medical organizations have been known to violate healthcare rights when it comes to keeping your job or giving accommodations. This is because historically the decision makers have been clinician leaders, who are often ignorant of the law. Only recently has this started to change, as organizations are now far more likely to have professional human resource managers.

Thus, should you find yourself dealing with a health issue, your first approach should not be to your department head or clinical boss who likely has no working knowledge of the law and health rights. Your first conversation should be with a disability or employment law attorney, and your second conversation should be directly with HR. Once you fully understand the legality of your health issue, only then should you approach your boss and colleagues. That conversation should be limited to facts and telling them legally what will be happening next.

11. Co-workers and administration

Perhaps this actually belongs in the previous chapter, because talking about co-workers or administration is really an issue of incivility. It can be so tempting to commiserate or adopt an us versus them attitude. There is so much that goes wrong in any given workday, it can be nice to have a scapegoat. Unfortunately, this type of gossip is a major driver of workplace toxicity, and you do not want to be seen as contributing to toxicity. Furthermore, you never really know who's side anyone is on in workplace politics.

12. Any highly polarizing contemporary event

As an experiment, right before writing this paragraph I opened up a major news website and scanned the stories. Trump versus Biden. Supreme court. De-criminalizing marijuana. Parental rights. Defund the police. Just to name a few . . .

It is tempting to talk about the zeitgeist. These are the major issues of our day, and most of us have a lot to say. Unfortunately, most of these will fall in our first eleven topics. Even when they do not, many contemporary issues have the same emotional and controversial qualities that undermine our ability to be rational speakers and receptive listeners.

New faces, new dangers

Having laid out these twelve pitfalls, it is not uncommon for someone to react by saying, "But I've talked about these things for years with my staff and partners, it was just that one time that went bad!"

There are a few reasons why this might have been. Perhaps these conversations weren't actually as well received as you thought they were all along. With increased social accountability and the introduction of formal HR practices into the world of medicine, it may just be that someone finally felt comfortable to speak up. Also, remember the professional verses unprofessional diagram in Chapter Five? It is dynamic and what was acceptable (or at least ignored) even just a few years ago no longer is.

Another reason why things may have gone awry despite years of engaging in the same type of conversation is due to *new faces:*

> *Erik was an ENT physician in a small private practice for the last 9 years. He loved going to work, in large part because of the people. It was a casual environment, where many people knew each other outside of work as well,*

especially through church. As such, conversations around religion, current events, and family were common.

However, many of the long time staff were starting to retire, creating staffing issues. It was also becoming increasingly difficult to survive financially as a small, unaffiliated practice. As a result, the practice was sold to a large, local healthcare system. The system brought in a clinic manager, and nurses from other practices in the system started cross-covering to ensure adequate staffing.

Not soon thereafter, some of those same nurses started reporting feeling uncomfortable in Erik's practice. Within six months, Erik was approached by the administration for "boundary issues" and creating a hostile work environment.

Erik's story is incredibly common. Historically, many of us have practiced in environments that were very stable in terms of people. Turnover was low, we worked with the same people for a long time, and there was a lot of self-selection in terms of who worked where. As a result, those people knew us and we knew them. We likely had a lot in common. If we said something that upset someone, we had years of positive interactions to offset that experience allowing the other person to assume good will and give us the benefit of the doubt (or at least be more inclined to forgive).

In fact, this is research proven. The same researchers mentioned above, Young and Saxe, also found if we don't know someone well, we don't trust them. When we don't trust them, we are far less likely to give their intent any weight as a mitigating factor when taking issue with something that they said. In contrast, when we know someone well, we weigh intent far more heavily and are more likely to assume there is some good will behind what they said.

So with this in mind, how many people at work do you not know well these days? A lot I imagine. Medicine is increasingly a multidisciplinary team sport. Consolidation of practices has resulted in large systems where people are moved around as needed. Chronic staffing shortages have fueled a massive increase in the use of locums workers. As such, we are often interacting with people we don't know well and have no track record with. Our colleagues are increasingly more likely to have trained elsewhere, experienced different work cultures, and have less in common with us. This all dramatically decreases trust and increases the likelihood of a communication or boundary violation.

And remember it doesn't even have to be the person we are interacting with. It is enough that the new face may simply overhear the conversation and take offense.

Listening as the best defense

Given all of this, the best defense is obviously to avoid certain conversation topics, both in talking with others but even when referring to ourselves. Furthermore, we need to avoid the urge to "doctor" by helpfully jumping into a conversation we are overhearing. But what about when the other person engages with us on one of these topics? How can deftly navigate that challenge?

One option may simply be to shut down or bow out of the conversation. For example, if someone is trying to engage with you in a way that is clearly a poor topic (their sexual exploits this last weekend, for example), it is perfectly reasonable to say, "I just don't think that is an appropriate topic for here and now."

You may, however, want to be a bit more gentle in your opting out. For example, if a person is really passionate to talk about politics or religion you may want to deflect more lightly. It may be enough to just say, "Thats an important (or interesting) topic, and I am not going to be able to give it the thought and attention it deserves at this moment." Or, "Maybe we should talk about that at another time in another setting more appropriate for the deep level of conversation it deserves."

But what if they just insist, and there is no deft way out? In this case, listening is the best defense. It is possible to have a whole conversation with someone that feels very meaningful to them without actually saying anything yourself. This involves a three-prong strategy of *listening, acknowledging, and validating*.

So listening is just that, really listen. Ignore the "doctoring" instinct to jump in, comment on, or problem solve. Then while listening you need to also acknowledge, which is really just showing them you are hearing what they are saying. This involves parroting back what they are saying, using soft language:

- It sounds like . . . [paraphrase what they said]
- It seems like . . .
- What I am hearing is . . .
- So you are saying. . . .

The use of this language is key. It makes people feel very heard without you actually having to agree, disagree, or add additional thoughts to the conversation.

Last, you want to validate how they feel. Again, soft language is key. You never want to say, "I know how you feel," or "I totally get that," because you really don't. That type of language can actually come across as condescending or agreeing - neither of which you want to do. Rather, you can simply say:

- I imagine that must be . . [tough, sad, hard, etc]
- That sounds incredibly . . .
- I can see you feel really strongly about this feeling of . . .

The power of the Listen-Acknowledge-Validate paradigm is you don't have to agree with someone's content to acknowledge what they are saying and validate how they feel. For example, imagine you have a male colleague who is the only male in an all female division, and he is criticizing administration for what he feels is sexist behavior. You disagree and feel that you have not seen anything to that effect. You realize that this is a high-risk conversation where you could easily misstep, negate his experience, and come across as sexist yourself. You also realize that if you fake agreement out of politeness and commiserate that could be interpreted as incivility towards the organization. It is a lose-lose.

So you just listen. You acknowledge and validate. You use statements like, "It sounds like you have felt treated differently as a male on multiple occasions, I imagine that is hard to feel that way when you come to work." Parrot what you heard, acknowledge how they *feel*.

It sounds simple, but the conversational impact can be profound. The other person often feels very validated and listened to. At the same time, you are not actually being sucked into the content of the conversation. You are unlikely to say anything that will be misinterpreted because you are not really saying anything. Also, your validation of how someone feels is not the same as agreement with their interpretation. You can thus use this technique even when you adamantly disagree with someone's perspective.

This technique is not just for the workplace, either. Try it with your partner or children. You will be surprised at the power of just listening!

Having an outlet

I will close this chapter by saying that while these topics are not appropriate for work, it is important to talk about them *somewhere*. It is human nature to want to talk about what is happening in our world right now. Also, we are intellectuals. As such we enjoy debate and tough conversations. Therefore, it is key that you do have some kind of outlet.

The problem for many physicians is that when you work 60 hrs a week (plus another 10-20 hrs of uncompensated duties like after-hours charting, emails, putting out fires, etc), it can be hard to have another outlet. When work is all you do, it *has* to be your everything. It has to be the place where you vent, flirt, get validation, talk about the zeitgeist, complain about your in-laws, talk about money, etc. Unfortunately, *it can't be any of those things.* So you need a place where this can happen with like-minded individuals. In other words, you need some sliver of a social life.

CHAPTER SEVEN

No Touching!

The perils of therapeutic touch

Thus far the majority of what we have talked about is verbal behavior, but what about touch? Perhaps more than any other chapter in this book, I have been looking forward to writing this one. That is because I knew it was going to be so simple and straightforward. When it comes to touching others:

DON'T.

(End of chapter.)

Unless you are performing a physical exam on a patient, your hands should never touch another human being at work regardless of whether they are a colleague or patient. It is just too risky. It is too easy for a benign touch to be interpreted as intimate, hostile, or anywhere in between.

Take a lesson from Keanu Reaves

Yes, that Keanu Reeves. For those who need a reminder, Mr. Reeves is an international superstar who starred in movies such as Speed and The Matrix. He also has an almost cult-like reputation for being a generous, self-aware, and humble guy - so much so that he holds the title of "The Internet's Boy-friend." One often-cited reason for why he is thought of as such a stand-up person is that he never touches another person (fan or celebrity) when he poses with them for pictures. Although it appears as if he puts his arm around their waist or on their back, he actually hovers his hands an inch or two away from them.

Now when I first heard about Keanu's "hover hands" I was skeptical, but it is indeed true and well documented. So consider that for a moment. Keanu Reeves is an A-list celebrity and international sex symbol. Not only would most people not mind if he touched them, I am willing to bet there are millions of people out there who explicitly want to be touched by him. So if *he* thinks twice about touching people, SO SHOULD YOU!

If Keanu isn't enough to convince you, you should also realize that virtually all healthcare organizations have an employee conduct policy that states it is never acceptable to touch another employee for any reason. These are zero tolerance policies written in black and white, and thus no mitigating circumstances are considered a reasonable defense. Now if your colleague collapsed in cardiac arrest in the middle of a hallway and you did chest compressions they *might* be willing to look the other way, but that is just about the only scenario in which they will.

Be careful around patients, too!

Touching patients is obviously unavoidable. The white coat allows us certain liberties with other peoples' bodies that are unimaginable to most lay people. Nonetheless, we must take great care. Any exam involving sexualized areas of the body needs to be done with a chaperone. This is just as true if you are performing it on a patient of the same gender. Likewise, particularly sensitive conversations, especially of sexual nature should be had with someone else in the room. And before you say that it is too much of an inconvenience to have to find someone to chaperone you every time, think of much of an inconvenience it is to lose your privileges or end up with an NPDB report against you!

Now I realize that for some of us, this might all seem extreme. Depending on where you grew up, when you when to medical school, as well as other cultural factors, touch may be an important part of how you conduct yourself. You may not hesitate to put a hand on a patient's shoulder in a difficult moment. Or you may naturally be physically affectionate with colleagues (pat on the back, hug, etc). You might not think twice about doing an unchaperoned hernia exam on a male as a male yourself. Unfortunately, you put your career in extreme peril when you do these things. My only advice is don't.

I told you this chapter would be short.

"e-" Stands for "Evidence"

Social media, electronic communications, and EHR

Lindsey was two weeks into her PGY-5 surgical year. She was widely regarded as one of the program's top residents. She was going to have her pick of any fellowship she wanted. One night on trauma service she operated on a very complicated case. She personally performed much of the surgery, with her attending watching dutifully. No other resident would have been given quite so much free rein, but again, she was exceptional. After closing the abdomen she took a photo with her cell phone. All you could see in the picture was a row of staples, there weren't really even any anatomic landmarks to say if this was the abdomen, the back, or the thigh. She posted it on one of her social media pages with a caption that simply said, "So proud of my hardest case to date, definitely saved this woman's life last night."

A few days later she was called into the GME office. She was shown the photo and asked if she took it, to which she said, "Yes." The head of GME then explained to her that because her social media page indicated where she worked, people could reasonably deduce where this case occurred. Furthermore it was date and time stamped narrowing down when the case occurred. The use of "this woman's life" in her caption also indicated

gender. Those things, combined with metadata within the photo file, rep-
resented multiple HIPPA protected elements. Furthermore, her
institution had a strict policy against the use of personal devices to record
audio or video content on campus. She was terminated immediately and
never found another residency spot to continue her training.

The threats to our livelihood from poor choices regarding social media, electronic communications, and EHR cannot be overstated. Social media in
particular tends to get us in trouble two ways. First, it is too easy to violate
HIPPA as the above example shows. Second, social media has a disinhibiting
effect not unlike alcohol. Email and texting also put us at constant risk of
being misunderstood because they can be taken in a way other than they were
intended.

Social media and HIPPA

We all know that patients have a right not to have their personal health information shared. What most of us don't realize, however, is how easy it is to
violate this through a simple social media comment. First of all, there are 18
data identifiers that are considered part of HIPPA. Some of these, such as
name or social security number, we intuitively realize cannot be shared. However, there are many other data elements that we may not think twice about.
For example, almost *any* date related to the person (admission date, discharge
date, date of procedure, date of death) is considered HIPPA. Therefore, like
our friend Lindsey above, simply implying the date of a procedure or an admission through a social media post (all of which are time/date stamped) can
be a violation. Diagnoses are also protected, so saying "I saw an awesome collapsed lung last night," can be a violation depending on what other
information might be available or implied on your account. Gender is also

protected, so simply using gendered pronouns inadvertently conveys information. The point is this: it is truly almost impossible to post a comment or thought about a patient without creating a potential violation.

Video and photos have even more risk. Even if the photo or video has no face or other identifying information, it likely still bleeds HIPPA information. Background objects, other people in the photo, and of course your comments may make it very easy to narrow down factors about the patient. Even if you are certain these aren't present, the file of the photo contains metadata, including date and time of creation and the GPS coordinates of where the photo was taken - often sufficient enough for a violation.

Also, your organization/hospital likely has a zero tolerance social media policy that is even more stringent than HIPPA. Pictures and video are likely never allowed for any reason, and poor behavior on social media is likely grounds for *termination with cause*. Also, most hospitals are very proactive about protecting HIPPA and enforcing their policies. Every organization I have worked with has people whose job it is is to surveil social media. They actively search the internet using the names of current employees as well as looking for hashtags related to the organization. If you post something on Facebook, LinkedIn, Tik Tok or the like, someone will find it.

Social media and disinhibition

The powers that be will also be scrutinizing your social media for more than just HIPPA. They will be scrutinizing your activity for anything that may reflect poorly on you as a professional or the organization as a whole. This includes:

- Disparaging comments about the organization or culture
- Disparaging comments about patients
- Disparaging comments about peers

- Medical misinformation or views significantly deviating from standards of care
- Any semblance of unethical behavior

The problem here is really one of disinhibition. Our personal filters for some reason do not work well in the world of social media. The barriers to engaging with social media are almost non-existent, and no one vets our content before we hit "send." Any moment of any day we can pick up our phone and get an immediate sense of gratification which is almost addictive. Furthermore, it feels very anonymous and safe as we fire off missives into the electronic ether.

As a result, we tend to be very disinhibited when engaging with social media - we say things and criticize in a way that we would never would be willing to do face-to-face.

Marcus was a pulmonary/critical care fellow at a large academic institution. He had always posted on social media since the beginning of medical school, often discussing his medical training journey but always careful to never talk about patients or his organization.

Halfway through Marcus's first year in fellowship, COVID hit. Like most of his peers, he saw more death and morbidity than he ever imagined. He could only watch in horror while his ICU and hospital basically collapsed from patient volume. He also became increasing frustrated at the politicization of COVID and masking, as well as at the families of critically ill patients who were COVID deniers. His social media posts increasingly reflected these frustrations and he tried to educate people through his online content.

In response to one of his more popular posts he was contacted by the local newspaper who wanted to interview him. He saw this as a great way to get some reliable information out there. He was interviewed on a wide range of topics related to COVID.

Unfortunately, the article that went to press was much more focused on the politics of COVID. The article left out 90% of what he was interviewed about, and focused on some of his quotes about anti-vaxxers, patients' families, and certain political groups.

A few days later Marcus was called into HR. While nothing he said was medically or statistically incorrect, the organization felt that his comments were unprofessional and condescending towards a few groups - groups which made up a significant part of the organization's revenue base. Marcus was suspended for 1 week and required to take a professional boundaries and communication course.

Thus at a minimum, it is imperative to avoid comments about patients, peers, and your organization. However, that is probably not enough! Even if you do not mix your personal social media life and your professional life, you can still be fired for content wholly unrelated to your professional endeavors.

This happens every day to physicians and other healthcare providers. Just about any content that could be seen as "improper" or "conduct unbecoming" is enough. And who decides the moral high ground? Your organization or medical board, who likely scrutinizes you more than other professionals are scrutinized by their organizations. In fact, research shows that healthcare providers are in the top tier of professionals who get fired for social media content (along with law enforcement, teachers, media, and government officials - not surprising as these are all public-facing roles with high levels of responsibility and scrutiny).

While anything could be deemed an infraction, the common themes of posts resulting in administrative action for all professions are:

- Racism (28%)
- Workplace conflict (17%)
- "Bad jokes" and otherwise insensitive posts (16%)
- Acts of violence or abuse (8%)

- Discriminatory behavior/comments towards women or LGBTQ+ persons (7%)
- Politics (5%)

Now again, I am not telling you this to debate how organizations should or should not surveil social media. We could spend hours talking about how social media is an important tool for holding people accountable, unmasking abuses of power, and ensuring equity and democracy. We could also spend hours talking about how this creates a hidden system of surveillance that scares people into being compliant and self-governing citizen-employees who are expected to have no individuality or personal life.

But it doesn't matter which side of the debate you come down on. Rather, you need to know the perils. This is the system we live in.

Avoiding the social media trap

Fortunately, it is very easy to avoid the quicksand of social media. The recommendation is not all that different from the recommendation made in regards to physical touch. When it comes to social media:

DON'T.

For 95% of physicians, there is absolutely no professional reason to ever post anything related to your work on social media. It generally benefits no one, and it can only get you in trouble. There is nothing wrong with being on social media or even having a social media presence, it simply must remain completely isolated from your professional life. Also, great care must be taken to remember that even if what you are doing on social media has nothing to do with your professional life, it is still open to scrutiny.

For some, particularly those who grew up with social media, this can be a hard pill to swallow. Given how much time and energy we delicate to our professional work, to omit it from our online lives can feel false or incomplete. Also, if we are working 80 hours per week, there just isn't much else to share on social media. Nonetheless, the risks are simply too great. The safest course of action is curate a highly sterile representation of your life on social media and nothing more.

But what if social media is an important part of your business strategy?

There is a small percentage of physicians for whom a social media presence is necessary for their business. This usually occurs in elective specialities that focus on wellness and medical optimization. Examples include plastics, aesthetics, lifestyle/integrative medicine, obesity medicine, longevity medicine, sports performance medicine, etc. In these fields, social media may be a critical means of driving patients to the practice.

If this is true for you, you need a cohesive and legally-vetted social media strategy. Nothing should be posted without some form of a review process in place that scrutinizes the content for appropriateness and HIPPA. You should also have iron-clad, lawyer-generated releases for when a patient does allow HIPPA to divulged, such as for a testimonial or the use of before and after pictures.

Email, HIPPA-compliant messaging, and other e-nightmares

It is one thing to say to avoid social media, but what about the ubiquitous electronic communication that we cannot avoid using? Email and HIPPA-compliant text messaging services like Halo or Qliq are now an inescapable part of our daily work flow. Unfortunately, one major result of this technology is that while it has never been easier to communicate with people, the quality of communication has also never been worse. Email and text messaging should make our crazy, multi-tasking, and team-oriented work days easier, but they also have the potential for miscommunications and frustrations that never used to exist.

One of the biggest problems with electronic communication is that it lacks the cues that we rely on when speaking in person. We can't see another person's face or body language through email. We can't hear the tone of their voice in a text. Neither can they ours. Without this non-verbal context, it is so easy for an email or text to come across abrasive, passive-aggressive, or dismissive; whereas if we had said the exact same thing in person there might not have been a problem.

A second massive problem with electronic communications is that they actually are not nearly as helpful or efficient as we expect them to be.

Douglas was a nephrologist whose group covered two hospitals. The call schedule was such that the person on call would work a full clinic day, take call at night, and still have clinic the next day.

One night a nurse paged him at 2am with the patient's latest BMP and low urine output. She was wondering how she should adjust the IV fluids. Douglas needed more information, so he texted back requesting full ins-and-outs as well as a few other labs. The nurse by that time had been pulled into another room, and couldn't get back to him until 2:45. That resulted in a few more back and forth texts until 3:15. Getting a little frustrated Douglas ultimately asked her to read the consult note from the day as it covered everything she was asking about, and he provided a recommendation for the fluids. Just as Douglas finally fell back asleep, the pager went off at 3:50 waking him up again. It was the same nurse just texting a sincere "thank you."

Not surprisingly, Douglas was overtired and frustrated the next day. So was the nurse, who felt he had been condescending and curt in a few of his replies.

e-strategies

So how do we navigate this quagmire of interconnectedness? Well, in the case of social media, the strategy as mentioned above is to disconnect. Social media is only downside when it comes to the professional domain of your life.

Now with e-communications disconnection is not possible, but we can mitigate the potential for miscommunication by knowing when not to e-communicate. Take the example of Douglas above, and think for a moment how would this have played out not that long ago. First, getting a hold of Douglas would have required calling him at home. As such, the conversation on the phone would have taken 5 minutes, not two hours of slow text back and forth. All lab data could have been asked for and immediately given, they could have discussed next steps in decision making as well as anticipated contingencies, and the tone of each person's voice would have assured the other that each was doing his or her best to help the other.

So one solution is therefore to take these conversations off-line. Texting and email are great for asking simple questions or providing a single piece of information. The moment things are more complex than that, it is better to speak directly. So once you realize there is any complexity, simply text back, "this sounds complex, please call me at ext 0900." Had Douglas done that with the initial text, he probably could have been back asleep by 2:30 instead of 4am, with a conversation that was more satisfying to both parties.

Similarly, once you realize you are having back and forth conversations by email, or a topic is complex or emotionally charged, switch to in-person communication as well. Ultimately, it will save you time and more importantly there is far less potential for misunderstanding your intent.

When you do choose to / have to communicate electronically, it can also help to keep the following guidelines in mind:

- Never send an electronic communication while emotional. If you felt catharsis, righteousness, or cleverness upon finishing an email or text, Do NOT send it (writing it was probably more about your control agenda than being beneficent to the other)
- If you wouldn't say it directly to someone's face exactly the way its worded in your text or email, don't say it electronically
- NEVER CAPITALIZE WORDS for emphasis - it will be interpreted as hostile / yelling
- Never engage in personal communications using a work-based device
- If you don't want the world to see what you've written, don't use electronic communication

This last bullet point is particularly important. As any lawyer will tell you, the "e-" in e-mail stands for *evidence.* You can never take back something sent electronically. All email and HIPPA-compliant text solutions are archived for years. If a subject is delicate, complex, or fraught with medico-legal implications, you need to be having face-to-face conversations with no electronic paper trail.

Information everywhere - EHR

Last, we would be remiss if we did not address EHR. The EHR gives us unfettered access to incredible amounts of information. Our accessing of this information is watched every moment of everyday.

Now most of us are clear on the idea that we should never access the clinical information of someone who we don't have a direct professional care responsibility for as a physician. Looking up what happened to that famous person just admitted to our hospital, for example, is a very quick way to get fired.

But it is easier to err than you might think:

Jack was an opthomologist at a major academic center. For weeks his wife had been asking him to provide the addresses of a few colleagues so that she could send out their Christmas party invitations. One Friday at 4:30pm, she called Jack at work saying she was at the post office and needed those addresses now.

Jack knew there was a faculty directory he had access to, but did not know off the top of his head how to get to it. He was, however, already logged into the EHR. Knowing that all employees are in the EHR for occupational health purposes, he accessed the demographics info of a few colleagues. He thought this would be ok because 1) he did not actually enter the clinical portion of their chart, and 2) this was information the university gave him access to through other means.

About a week later, IT contacted him requesting an explanation as to why he accessed those charts, which he provided. Not soon after HR recommended to the Medical Executive Committee that he be terminated. The MEC reviewed the incident, and ultimately choose to clinically suspend him 5 weeks. He was also required to undergo remedial education regarding HIPPA and EHR as well as provide a Grand Rounds lecture on what he learned.

Due to the length of the suspension, this triggered an automatic report to the National Provider Data Base (NPDB), which in turn generated an automatic report to the state medical board. They conducted their own investigation resulting in a "Public Letter of Concern" that was now searchable by all future employers, insurers, and patients.

The above case reveals two common mistakes that I have seen many times. First, any access of the EHR, even when *clinical* information is not accessed, is considered access that requires a patient-doctor relationship to be justified. Second, I have seen many physicians err by assuming that accessing the record was justified because it was information that they were otherwise allowed to have through another mechanism (ex: faculty directories, research data sets, etc).

This can even be true of our own medical information! For example, there are employers that do not allow providers to access their own charts through the EHR ever. In these organizations, employees are not allowed to log in to the EHR and access their own chart to see the same results that they are allowed to see by logging in as a "patient" through the online patient portal!

In contrast, some organizations do allow you to view your own patient data using the EHR. However, there are often strict rules that you cannot alter the chart in any way or engage in any care. For example, you may realize that an important allergy is not listed in your chart. Putting that allergy in would be a violation of organizational rules. Similarly, if you needed one of your nurses to place a TB test on you for your annual occupational health compliance, ordering it yourself would likely be an infraction. Documenting the result yourself would also likely be an infraction.

As you can see, the EHR is a minefield. Make sure you absolutely have a clear and *active* doctor-patient relationship with the person whose data you are accessing. Outside of having this, do not access data through the EHR even if you have access to that same data through other means. Last, know your organization's rules regarding EHR and your own personal data.

———————

As you can see, a theme is emerging. Social media is not our friend. Electronic communications are not the efficient panacea that our administrators pretend that they are. EHR will bite you in the ass. Don't be seduced by their relative ease! Stay off social media. Engage in face-to-face or voice-to-voice communication when dealing with anything complex or significant, as it is safer and often more efficient.

CHAPTER NINE

Disruptive Advocacy

Conflict and advocacy communication skills

So much of what we have touched upon so far is what *not* to say and what *not* to do. The previous chapters were primarily about building self-awareness around common pitfalls and developing skills for avoiding them. But what about when we need to engage in friction? How do we address problems and advocate without without being seen as a problem?

One of the biggest challenges for physicians I work with who have been through an administrative process is that once they are under a PIP or PHP contract, they feel completely disempowered. As a result, when a patient or family member is being unreasonable, they are afraid to exert proper bound-aries (ex: refusing to prescribe antibiotics) because the patient might then file a complaint. They don't know how they can approach a colleague about that person's problematic behavior because they are afraid that the colleague can turn it around on them and say that they were uncivil or belligerent. After all, who is administration going to believe? Physicians don't know how to push back on administration and advocate for improvements without being further labeled "disruptive."

Thus in this chapter we are going to address practical skills for each of these scenarios. In doing so, some common themes will emerge. I would argue that rather than memorizing these scripts, its more important to understand why these scripts work - i.e. what are the underlying emotional needs that are being addressed and how do these techniques address those needs? Once you understand that, you will have the artistic freedom to deploy these skills in just about any scenario and alter them as necessary to fit the situation.

First, understand that every conversation is crucial

Crucial Conversations by Joseph Grenny is a well-known bestselling book on interpersonal communication. In it the author notes that most communication breakdown occurs when a conversation is "crucial." He defines crucial conversations as those having three elements:

- Opposing opinions
- High stakes
- Strong emotions

Unfortunately, almost every interaction in medicine can easily meet these criteria. Stakes are always high so that is just a given. If our opinions or perspectives weren't opposing, we probably wouldn't be conversing to begin with. What tends to be variable is the amount of emotion both parties are bringing to the conversation. This is why so much of the focus of this book so far has been about introspection and emotional self-regulation. The problem is that even when we are very skilled in this regard, the people around us are often emotionally activated due to chronic stress. Therefore, we need to be constantly vigilant and bring these skills to bear in every conversation because the only variable that we can really control is the emotionality of the interaction. With that idea in mind, we will explore three scenarios.

The upset patient (EASY protocol)

While this technique can work for anyone coming to you upset, we use the example of a patient because that is one we are all very familiar with. We have all walked into a room where you can immediately cut the tension with a knife. Or we have had an interaction that seemingly started off well, but suddenly takes a turn.

In either of these scenarios, it is first important to understand *your* tendency in these situations. Remember cognitive and emotional avoidance? It applies here as well. We don't like when others are upset. It is emotionally uncomfortable and we *reactively* want to get rid of that emotion one way or another (notice the problem is not the conflict itself, but our desire to avoid our internal discomfort with it!). As such, when we sense that someone else is upset, we tend to react one of two ways - with *silence* or *violence*. This idea, again from the book *Crucial Conversations*, is that when faced with conflict we either pretend it isn't there or we immediately try to combat it.

For example, *silence* means we ignore the elephant in the room. The patient is upset, but we just plow through. We begin our history, do our exam, and push through the clinical encounter until we get out. Even though we know the patient is angry or upset, we don't address it if they don't (and they often won't - they just sit there seething).

The problem with this approach is that until the emotional bomb in the room is defused, the clinical encounter is pointless. How likely are they to be forthcoming in the history? How likely are they to put any stock in what you say or prescribe? Are they going to come back? You do manage to get out of the room without directly engaging in conflict this way, but at what cost in terms of actually helping the patient? How likely are they to stay silent in the room but then file a complaint later?

In contrast to silence, other physicians are more prone to *violence*. Now this does not mean hitting the patient! Rather, it refers to verbal combat and pushing back against the patient's emotionality - i.e., trying to negate or dismiss their position. Correcting them, trying to demonstrate why they should not be upset, or dismissing their feelings are all forms of violence. Focusing on defending yourself or others is a form of violence (i.e. prioritizing "looking good," and "being right"). Even problem solving can be a form of violence if it is more motivated by our desire to control (ie get rid of) our discomfort with having an upset patient in front of us (remember the control versus beneficence spectrum from Chapter Five?).

It is also important to note that you may have a tendency towards silence in certain scenarios, and a tendency towards violence in others. For example, many physicians tend towards silence when a patient or family is clearly upset. They don't want to engage and resort to being overly clinical in their interactions to avoid the emotional elephant in the room. Those same physicians, however, immediately resort to violence when a colleague comes to them aggressive or upset (for example, a feisty consult). They won't hesitate to attack first, push back, fight about who's right, etc.

Either way, these two tendencies are not effective. So instead of silence or violence, we want to find a middle way. We want to be *responsive* rather than reactive. Most importantly, we need to diffuse the other person's emotionality before we can proceed. To do this, we use the EASY protocol. EASY stands for:

- Empathize
- Apologize
- State the facts
- Find the Yes

<u>Empathize</u> - Not surprisingly, the first step in dealing with anyone who is emotional is empathize. Fortunately, we have discussed exactly how to do this using the Listen-Acknowledge-Validate strategy in Chapter Six. Once you realize someone is upset you must address that first, and just start listening. As previously discussed, don't interject or try to change minds, just listen.

Now what if they aren't talking but clearly upset? You have to make them talk. Once you sense something is off, you need to invite them to speak. "It seems like you are frustrated by something," or, "I get the sense you might be upset, will you tell me about it?" This kind of invitation is hard for those of us who have a tendency towards "silence." We have to overcome that, otherwise we will make no progress.

Now once they are talking you need to acknowledge and validate. You acknowledge what they are saying by parroting what they just said back to them, using soft language such as, "It seems that . . . ," or, "I'm hearing . . . " Then you validate, although here there is a slight difference than the type of validation we did in Chapter Six.

In Chapter Six, our goal was to validate their emotional state without committing to the content of what they were saying - for example, using language such as, "I am sorry you feel X, I imagine that is hard." We can use the same types of validation here, but there is a fine line between making them feel validated versus coming across as though we don't buy in to their concerns. Consider the following two validating statements:

> *"I'm sorry you thought that my body language was intimidating."*
> *vs.*
> *"I'm sorry you felt intimidated."*

The former statement could feel slightly condescending to the recipient because there is almost an implication that the interpretation of the body language is a problem with how the recipient is viewing the situation. There is almost a sense that perhaps someone else (i.e. someone more rational) would not have seen such body language as intimidating. Part of why this occurs is the use of the word "thought" rather than focusing on feelings. Another part of why this occurs is because there is mention of both "you" and "me" in the first statement, which almost juxtaposes the two.

In contrast, the later statement avoids this. It simply focuses on the other person and their feelings, and in doing so is likely to be heard as more sincere. So when making validating statements, avoid bringing yourself/others into the statement. Focus solely on the person's feelings and not their thought processes.

Apologize - At this point it is often reasonable to apologize. There is a good chance you may already have as part of your validation statements. Even so, it can be helpful to give a summative apology at this point. When apologizing, be specific. "I'm sorry," is fine, but "I am sorry that X and Y . . . " shows that you were really listening.

State the facts - Here is where things get a bit tricky. Although you have listened, acknowledged, validated, and apologized, you may still have to exert a boundary or give them information that they do not want to hear. This is where we may have to make an assertion. They key is we are making the assertion AFTER we have put their feelings first, defusing the situation a bit so that we can now have a rational conversation.

Now "the facts," i.e. your assertion, can take many forms. Perhaps you have to explain to them why something is the way it is. Perhaps you will have to explain why you won't be doing something. Maybe you have to correct their medical misunderstanding of something. Regardless, the strategy here is to say it as simply and factually as possible and avoid the use of a negating connective word when you move from the apology to your facts. Consider the following example:

"I am sorry you were not seen as soon as you were brought back to a room, but I was in another room with a very sick patient for longer than expected."

vs.

"I am sorry you were not seen as soon as you were brought back to a room. I was in another room with a very sick patient for longer than expected."

There is literally only one word difference between these two statements. Yet the "but" has a significant impact. When you use a negating connecting word, such as "but," "however," "nevertheless," "although," etc., it has the effect of discounting everything you say before it. You diminish the patient's experience or feelings, as well as your own preceding apology. This is why the second statement just works better. It makes space for both statements to be true and equally valid.

<u>Find the Yes</u> - Once you have asserted what you need to, its time to compromise. What can you do for the patient? How can you achieve some sort of resolution? Generally as the knowledge holder, it is up to you to come up with reasonable options for moving forward. "While I am not able to do X, I am able to do Y or Z." You can also ask the person for their input in terms of solutions depending on the situation. A very effective statement that I use often is, "Given that X is not possible, what *would* you like to have happen?" These types of open ended questions give the person in front of you the most autonomy. However, they can obviously backfire if the person then asks for impossible or unreasonable solutions. Thus this technique should be used with care.

Let's see EASY in action:

(E) It sounds like you've been though a lot going from provider to provider to figure out what is wrong with your knee. (A) I am sorry you were expecting to be able to get an MRI here today in the ER. (S) We do not

order MRIs from the ER as they are not used in diagnosing emergent sit-
uations. (Y) I would like to help you solve this. I can have my social
worker come in and talk to you. She has resources to help patients navigate
these challenges when they don't have insurance.

(E) If I am understanding you correctly, it sounds like you were called
and given one lab result that was normal, but later when you were look-
ing at your chart online the result was completely different and abnormal.
I imagine that was upsetting and confusing. (A) I am so sorry you had
that experience. (S) I honestly don't know how that happened. We have
safeguards in place to try to prevent that from happening, but those appear
to have failed. (Y) For my part, I am reporting this to my administration
so that we can figure out what happened. What else would you like to
have happen in terms of dealing with this result here and now?

So there you have it - EASY. Now that we have laid out the basics of the
structure, a few nuances are worth addressing. First, you may not always use
each part EASY or in the same order. *Empathize* always comes first, but after
that you may alter the structure depending on the specifics of the situation.
For example, when boundaries are really being pushed or someone is completely unreasonable, you may need to *state the facts* before apologizing. Also,
not all situations warrant an apology. It is also important to know that trying
to *"find the Yes"* may also result in emotions returning if finding a solution is
proving challenging, which may mean you have to go back to *Emphasize* and
run the cycle a few times to achieve a good outcome.

Confronting other's speech or behavior (STUN protocol)

Confronting others regarding their speech or behavior is in some ways the
opposite of the previous situation. In this scenario, you are likely the one who

is emotionally activated first, and you are the one to have to initiate the encounter. Furthermore, once you start to engage with the other person, they are likely to become emotionally activated and defensive (and they will likely move towards silence or violence). Thus the challenge is not that we have to first defuse the other person's pre-existing emotionality as in the scenario above; rather, we have to manage our own while not triggering the other person's as we engage. To do this, we use the STUN protocol:

- **S**tart with the facts
- **T**ell them the impact
- **U**ncover their perspective
- **N**eeds and goals

<u>Start with the facts</u> - Once you have found an appropriate time and place to talk, you want to start by factually outlining the speech or behavior that needs to be addressed. You want to be succinct and specific. Let's say you have a colleague who constantly makes comments behind patients' and employees' backs about their weight. You find it inappropriate and want this to stop. So when you start your discussion with that colleague, do not say, "You are always making rude comments about people's weight." He is likely to become defensive and will also likely try to prove you wrong by saying, "I don't *always* talk about people's weight."

Rather, say, "I wanted to talk about something you said. Today after we saw patient X, you commented on how she was 'too fat to wear that outfit.' Similarly, yesterday after lunch you joked about colleague X's weight gain after her pregnancy by saying [quote here]." You want to give concrete examples of the problem, ideally focusing on the most recent incidents even if it is a long standing pattern.

There are a few reasons we start with a specific and factual accounting of what occurred. First, you need to make sure the facts are agreed upon. If the other person doesn't even agree as to what was done or said, the rest of the conversation is moot. Second, by stating *just* the facts (and using quotes when possible), you are starting with the least debatable elements. This will minimize their ability to deny or deflect as the facts are facts. It will also help you start the conversation from a less emotionally charged place internally.

Tell them the impact - Once you have laid out a factual accounting of the behavior and the facts are agreed upon, you then start to provide your interpretation. You want to state how this behavior impacted your thoughts and feelings. In doing so, you want to keep the focus on yourself, using "I" language such as "When that happened, I felt X, and I thought Y." So instead of saying "*You* keep upsetting me by saying inappropriate comments," you can say, "When you said X and Y, *I* felt upset and *I* thought that it was inappropriate and rude. Also, as someone who used to be more overweight, it makes *me* wonder if I were heavier like I used to be how that would impact our professional relationship." Although this language difference might be subtle, it again makes it harder to become defensive because "I"-based language keeps the focus on the speech/action and its impact on you, rather than focusing more on the person doing it.

Uncover their perspective - If appropriate, this is where you solicit their thoughts and intent. The goal is to invite them to be open, with a focus on being generative. There are three great ways to do this:

- *Is that what you intended?*
- *Do you see it differently?*
- *Is there something I am missing here that would help me understand better?*

More often than not, you may be surprised by the answers. The offending person may simply have had no idea the impact of their behavior. If they value your relationship they will often apologize and actively try to change. Sometimes, you may discover that their intent was quite different, and their behavior may make much more sense from their perspective (although still problematic). You can then work together to come up with a better approach for getting both of your needs met. Or perhaps they have no valid explanation, or their viewpoint is still unacceptable to you after exploring it. That is fine. There is still utility in this step, as it allows the other to be heard which continues to diffuse emotion.

Needs and goals - Last, here is where you state what you need moving forward. Taking into account anything useful that you learned in Step Three, you now clearly state what you need to change. Again you want to be specific. What exactly must happen, how will you know that is happening, and when does it need to happen by? Also, what are the consequences of it not happening? "I need you to not make comments or jokes to me about people's weight. If you continue to do so I will [consequence]." This is also the section where you could problem solve together. Perhaps you don't have a clear sense of what should happen in response to a given situation, so here is where you try to come to some collaborative agreement.

As with the EASY protocol, the STUN protocol is about emotional management. Simply by having a plan with which to approach a difficult conversation you have more control, which in turn reduces your emotionality and allows you to communicate clearly. Second, the step-wise approach is designed to preemptively stun their becoming defensive, making them a better listener.

Now just as with the EASY protocol, you may not always use each step. However, it is always a good strategy to start with the facts for reasons discussed above. In the second step, however, you may choose to be less soft with your language when you tell them the impact depending on the egregiousness of the problem. Let's say someone made a rude comment about your body (and it wasn't the first time!). You will outline the facts using direct quotes, and then you very clearly tell them the impact. Also, since this a zero tolerance type of situation, there may be no need to solicit their perspective (after all, what perspective or mitigating factors could be valid?). Instead, you may simply go straight to *needs and goals*, outlining what must happen moving forward and the consequences for continued poor behavior.

The STUN protocol is great for any uncomfortable but crucial conversation where you need someone to do something differently moving forward.

Up-managing administration

Up-managing refers to how you navigate your relationships with supervisors and administrators (in contrast to those you oversee). It is a skill that physicians are never taught, which is a travesty given that it is now the case that over 50% of US physicians are employees of large healthcare organizations. So most of us now have bosses, so to speak. There are also more administrators that we must deal with than ever before. One study demonstrated that while the number of physicians grew 150% from 1975 to 2010, the number of healthcare administrators increased 3200% for the same time period.

Gone are the days where physicians took care of patients with little administrative oversight. We are now immersed in policies and procedures, reporting to non-clinical managers, metrics, and red tape. Unfortunately, what often happens is that physicians struggle with these ever-growing non-clinical aspects of their work. Not having a skillset with which to navigate these challenges, physicians often get frustrated, or worse, get labeled as disruptive.

Physicians and administrators are different species

To understand how we can better up-manage those around us, we need to first acknowledge the tremendous differences between our physician mission and the administrators that we are often dealing with. First, as physicians we focus helping the person sitting in front of us get what they need. In contrast, administrators focus on managing resources at a macro level. Likewise, we make individualized decisions patient by patient; administrators focus on broadly implemented systems-level change. We are medically trained; increasingly administrators are not.

We also make decisions and communicate very differently. In a clinical encounter, we often have no idea what we are walking to, and yet we quickly amalgamate vast sums of information and are expected to solve the problem in front of us in a matter of minutes (sometimes seconds!). We cut to the chase, seeing the solution in black and white and blurting it out. We do this alone and with little to no consensus. In contrast, administrators operate on a timeline of weeks to months to address a problem. Furthermore, they are taught to be "buy-in" seeking, often engaging in many meetings and conversations to tease out shades of grey before taking action.

Last, administrators lack the internalization of the patient's well-being that we discussed in Chapter Four. Simply put, administrators are not individually medically responsible for what happens to a patient, at least not in any binding legal sense. But we are. We therefore experience an emotionality and protectiveness with regards to patient care that administrators cannot appreciate. Combine this with everything mentioned above and you effectively have two totally different species of animal trying to work together. The potential for miscommunication is vast.

Stop trying to solve problems in meetings

Bearing all of these differences in mind, there are distinct strategies for dealing with administration when it comes to effecting change. The first is to realize that nothing meaningful has ever happened in a meeting. Meetings are often the only times when physicians are at the same table as mangers, thus physicians assume this is the time and place to get things done. In reality, as far as administrators are concerned, meetings are *pro forma* and *fait accompli*. The majority of meetings are where administrators present their conclusions and where they disseminate new policies under the guise of democracy.

Physicians, however, often do not understand this. Inevitably, there is always that physician with a pressing concern who thinks that when administrators ask at the end of a meeting, "Does anyone have anything else to bring up?" that they actually mean it. So that physician then opens a can of worms at :55 past the hour and tries to address something actually important. Inevitably they have to be cut off and told something like, "Thats a great topic for next time, let's all reflect on that," or, "Let's schedule another meeting for that."

Instead, its critical to realize that all the action happens in "pre-meetings." Pre-meetings are essential for addressing any challenge or contentious issue. These are small scale meetings, not always formal, often involving just a few people. If you have a concern or change you want to make, your first pre-meetings should be with peers to determine their assessment of the issue. Its always easier to face a challenge as a unified front, even if you are the main driver of the group. These early meetings are thus a time for coalition building and information gathering.

Next you expand and meet with other key players. You continue to build trust and rapport. You have an opportunity to try your ideas out on a wider group of people to see where the friction points are. You identify detractors and challenges while refining your approach. Thus by the time more formal meetings happen, most of the pieces are in place. You are bringing up an issue that everyone is aware of, and you have a well-articulated argument and proposed solution with people supporting you.

This last element - a solution - is particularly key. One of the most common mistakes physicians make is they are quick to identify problems but rarely have well-articulated solutions that are actually feasible to go with them. Physicians *vocalize*, but to be successful you need to engage in two-way communication and problem-solve. When you don't, all your vocalization does is add stress to your supervisor's already chronically overwhelmed mental state. You've given them another thing to deal with, and the most common response you will get is the supervisor deprioritizing your issue. Worse, you may be labeled "a problem" or disruptive.

This may sound cynical and condescending towards administrators, but it is backed by research. In a 2008 paper, researcher Jackie Macdonald analyzed the decision-making processes of healthcare administrators. She found that most administrators struggle to make decisions because they function in an environment where there are poorly-defined outcomes and significant time pressures. Furthermore, they often suffer from a lack of personal technical expertise. This results in a preference to assess the situation over and over rather than selecting a course of action, and a reliance on trying to make the current problem fit prior solutions rather than integrating new information and generating new ways forward.

So make it easy for them! Have a solution and have all of the pre-meetings necessary to get buy-in. Simplify the data, don't talk in shades of grey, and be straightforward. Also, make sure you understand what is important to them (i.e how are they assessed on their performance and by who?) and make sure you phrase things in those terms. Usually that means focusing on money and efficiency, not quality of care or provider well-being.

Make sure you are talking to the right people!

Another key to being successful is making sure that you are actually talking to the right people. Remember that the number of hospital administrators has increased by 3200% since 1975? That is true, but at the same time it is also true that the number of people with real power and decision-making abilities has *not* increased much at all. In any organization, real power is still limited to a few decision makers and the handful of people who have influence on those decision-makers.

To be blunt, this means that most administrators and supervisors are just middle men. Again, research supports this. Many studies have found that about 80% of managers in organizations add no real value to the organization and are not necessary or useful in any way. So you can have all of the conversations and pre-meetings you want, but unless they include one of the real decision-makers or their influencers, it's pointless. It is imperative that you find the decision-makers and influencers and strive to be someone that they can rely on to know what is really going on, provide good information, and generate solutions.

So the next time your immediate boss or department head starts talking about some potential changes and you need speak up and advocate for a certain outcome, find out who is really pulling the strings. Ask your boss, "Who asked you to look into this?" or, "Who will you go to with this information?" The answer to those questions is likely the real decision-maker. Once you identify that person, that is where your efforts should go. Why is this issue important to them, what outcomes do they care about? Even if you have to work through your immediate supervisor, at least then you can phrase things in ways that make sense to the person they ultimately have to report to.

Using a light touch

The last technique for up-managing, and perhaps the most important from a career-safety point of view, is using a light touch. As laid out above, we are critical thinkers with a well-refined ability to rapidly and bluntly shoot from the hip when there is a problem. We expect to be listened to as experts. This works well in many clinical situations, like a code, but again does us no favors in meetings when dealing with administrators. Many physicians have gotten in trouble not so much for what they said, but how they said it. This style of communication makes it too easy for administrators to label us "disruptive," when as far as we are concerned, we are being efficient, direct, and advocating for patients. To circumvent this, we need to revisit the idea of softening our language. We touched upon this in Chapter Six and now we will explore more techniques for doing so. The first such technique is using open-ended questions.

Of everything I have learned in my years of coaching and having difficult conversations with people, the power of open-ended questions has been the most useful. An open-ended question is a question that cannot be answered in "yes" or "no." For example, "Do you think this change will impact patient safety?" is a closed-ended question whereas, "How do you think this change will impact patient safety?" is an open-ended question.

The power of open-ended questions is that they force a generative answer. In doing so, they have multiple effects. First, it forces the person to further reveal their thinking, which can be helpful for you during any contentious conversation. Second, it allows you to bring up disagreement and make your own points without actually having to bluntly say that you disagree.

Consider the following example: you are in a meeting and the OR manager is proposing a new process for room turnover between cases. It is clearly aimed at reducing cost, but as an anesthesiologist you can immediately see that this will prolong time between cases, increase your work, and potentially undermine patient-safety processes previously put in place.

It is not uncommon that a physician will respond by saying, "That is a bad idea! Clearly this is a cost-saving measure with no regard for patients or providers. By no longer doing X, we are skipping a patient-safety process that has long been in place, and that is clearly stupid and we are all going to get sued. Second, . . . "

Again, blunt and to the point, but in today's environment that kind of response will be labeled as disruptive. It creates animosity rather than teamwork. So what if we rephrased it with open-ended questions? For example, "I can see the cost-saving benefits of X and Y with this new procedure. But I am curious, how are we going to implement this without undermining patient-safety mechanism Z?"

The beauty of this approach is rather than telling them your point, you are forcing *them* to articulate your own point. They have to answer the question, and in doing so, one of a few things will happen. First, maybe they did not realize the problem in the first place. Now they do and it must be addressed. Another possibility is that they knew there was a problem and tried to ignore it. Now they are called out on it. If they try to BS their way through a solution, or dismiss the problem outright, they will have to do it verbally and in front of the whole group.

The best part, however, is that no one can label you disruptive. They may get very flustered at your question, but as long as you pretend to be curious and say it with a smile, they cannot say that you were blaming, judgmental, or disruptive. Feigned curiosity is the antidote to being labeled a problem-maker.

And one last subtle point in regards to open-ended questions: avoid the use of the word "why." In coaching we have a saying, "Who, what, when, where, how, but NEVER why." The reason is that "why" tends to put people on the defensive. Although it is technically an open-ended question, it is the least soft of the open-ended options. Fortunately, an easy solution is to just substitute "how" any time you find yourself about to ask a "why" question. For example, compare the following:

> *Why do you think that is true?*
> *Why do you think this is the best option?*
> *vs.*
> *How do you know that is true?*
> *How did you decide this was the best option?*

The first two questions using "why" are simply more abrasive. By substituting "how" and feigning curiosity you can raise the same concern and demand the same response in a softer way.

In this chapter we have covered a wide range of communication techniques. Again, you can memorize these as scripts. I would argue, however, that it is better to understand the underlying reasons why these techniques work. In a word, it all comes down to emotionality. We manage our own emotions by knowing how we might get hooked and by having a plan for communication. We manage other's emotionality by perspective-taking, acknowledging and validating their feelings, and using soft language. The best communicators are those most comfortable with emotion when it shows up. They do not move towards silence or violence, but rather embrace whatever is coming head on, and deftly work with it to achieve a positive resolution.

CHAPTER TEN

Restorative Processes

Is punishment the only way to repair?

Most of the physicians I work with tell me that one of the most challenging aspects of going through a disciplinary process is the inability to make amends to the person(s) harmed. Once a physician is able to take the other person(s) perspective and understand why their own speech or behavior was problematic, they often want to somehow make it right.

Yet what usually happens is that the physician is explicitly told not to bring up the issue or engage in any conversation with anyone, especially with the harmed party. Interaction with the harmed person(s) is to be kept at the minimum required for direct patient care. At the same time, those harmed are not allowed to know what corrective actions have been taken. For example, they have no idea that the physician is under a PIP, taking a communications course, or working with a coach.

The result of all of this is that the physician undergoes a disciplinary process *today*, and is often right back at work with the harmed person(s) *tomorrow*. The physician has no ability to make amends, and those harmed do not see that any action was taken. The relationship remains damaged, and yet these people now have to work together with patients' lives in the balance. This is not satisfactory to either party involved, nor is it in the best interest of the organization.

A better way?

We would be better served doing something in leiu of, or in addition to, punishment and corrective action. One option is "restorative justice." Restorative justice is often discussed in the context of criminal behavior, but restorative processes are applicable to any situation in which one person has harmed another or a relationship has been damaged.

Restorative processes recognize that in these types of situations, all the people involved have psychological needs. The people who were harmed often need to feel safe again, which generally means they need to feel that this situation won't recur. They want the other person to know how they were harmed, and how they felt. They also often want to understand the other person's motivations or what led to this harm occurring.

Likewise, the person who did the harming also has psychological needs. They often want to apologize and be able to offer amends. They want to feel that this one incident won't solely define them moving forward. They often want to express the thoughts behind their actions. When possible, they want to restore the relationship.

With these psychological goals in mind, this chapter will explore what a restorative process looks like, and how you might participate in such a process in order to repair your relationships.

Now at this point, you might be asking why isn't this chapter at the beginning of the book? Isn't this something that should have happened early on? Perhaps. In most scenarios a restorative process is most effective if it happens soon after the incident (although allowing some time for cooler minds to prevail). However, as you will see, the successful navigation of a restorative process will require many of the insights and tools discussed in the preceding chapters. In a sense, restorative processes build upon everything else we have touched upon. Therefore we present it now, after all of the other hard work you have done.

Punitive Processes	Restorative Processes
Poor speech/behavior violates rules	Poor speech/behavior violates relationships
Focus on guilt	Focus on needs and responsibilities
Applies punishment / corrective actions	Makes things "right"
Adversarial process	Agreement through dialogue
Administration is central	Victim and offender are central
Rules are key	Assumption of responsibility is key
Win/lose outcomes	Needs met and healing on both sides
Community members are separated	Community members are brought together
Focus on past	Focus on future

First, some major warnings!

If this far into the book you still do not feel that you had any culpability in what happened, or you cannot see the other person's perspective and how they were harmed, *do not participate* in an attempt at a restorative process. A fundamental pillar of restorative processes is that you are able to acknowledge responsibility for the negative impact that you created, and that you are able to acknowledge any harm caused (even if that harm was not intended). If you go into this process with goals like convincing others of your version of "truth," being right and looking good, or getting the other person to apologize, you are likely to do more harm than good.

Second, DO NOT ATTEMPT A RESTORATIVE PROCESS ON YOUR OWN! Do not attempt to pull the person with whom you have had conflict aside to "have a talk." Don't corner them in the cafeteria. Do not write, email, or call them no matter how well-meaning you are. Any of these could upset the other person, be perceived as intimidating, and make a bad situation worse. If you wish to try a restorative process, it must be brokered through a third-party such as HR or clinical administration. Although it may be at your request, they should take the lead in making sure that all parties are willing to participate without coercion. They should create the safe space in which to have these conversations, and they should provide mediation / structure. If they are not willing to do so, do not attempt to force the issue through some other means.

The five R's

Assuming you are able to participate in a restorative process, you want to do everything you can to maximize its effectiveness. To do this you will need address each of the five R's - *relationship, respect, responsibility, repair, and re-integration.*

Relationship - For your part in the process, you want to make it clear to others that your concern is the relationship that has been harmed. At the beginning, consider talking about that relationship and why it is important. How is the other person(s) central to care of the patient and your ability to do your job? Acknowledge that you may spend more time interacting with this person than you do with your partner or other family members. Given that, your day-to-day relationship with this person(s) has a significant impact on your well-being. Also, spend some time talking about what your relationship looks like when it is at its best. Doing all of this sets the stage for why this process is important and clarifies your intent and goals.

Respect - Conveying respect during this process is paramount. The best way to do that is with deep, active listening. The other person needs to feel heard and respected (even if you disagree at times). Their point of view must be honored.

To do this well, we can borrow from the *listen, acknowledge, and validate* process in Chapter Six. First and foremost, just listen. Do not interject, add, or correct when they are talking about their interpretations or experiences. You also want to make it clear that you are not just listening, but *hearing*. Acknowledging through repeating back what you are hearing makes sure that you are in fact hearing correctly, and the other person now has proof that you heard.

Lastly, you need to validate their experience. Now here is where we will diverge a bit from the type of validation used in Chapter Six. In Chapter Six we were specifically trying not to validate the content of what someone was saying; rather, we were trying to validate only the emotions. The problem is, if we do this now we can come across as if we do not believe them.

For example, you engaged in incivility during a consult. Your wording and tone could have been much better. While listening to the person you upset, you try to validate what they are saying one of two ways:

> *"I am sorry you found my wording upsetting during the consult."*
> *vs.*
> *"I am sorry I upset you."*

Which sounds more sincere? In the first instance, one could argue that culpability might be shifted, ie., it's the harmed person's problem that they "found my wording upsetting." The implication is that maybe someone else would not have. In other words, this phrasing puts the focus on the harmed person's interpretation, rather than the fact that harm was caused. Thus when validating in this instance (versus the scenarios in Chapter Six), it is important to validate not just the emotional content but also validate their point of view and interpretation.

Responsibility - You have to take responsibility for your part in the process. Every participant will be asked to make a critical self-appraisal and search for any way they might have contributed to the situation, even if not intentionally. However, this does not mean that you should expect others to feel responsible so that you can feel less responsible. This is not about what others can give to you, only what you can give to them.

Another aspect of responsibility is being willing to give an explanation of what may have caused your behavior. This is tricky, because you must be very diligent not appear to shirk responsibility by blaming others or the system. At the same time, there are often are factors at play that may not have been obvious to others (or even yourself) at the time of the incident. Knowing these can inform the next step in the process - repair.

Repair - It is important to recognize that punishment is not repair. You may feel quite punished. Perhaps you were suspended or required to spend money on a corrective course or therapist. These requirements, however, do not directly repair the relationship with the person you harmed, especially given that they are unlikely aware of your punishment. Keeping this in mind can help prevent the unproductive mindset of, "I've already lost so much time and money in this process, and had my name dragged through the mud, what more could you possibly want?"

How can amends be made? How can underlying factors be eliminated or mitigated? This part of the process is about both direct repair to the person harmed and also repairing contributing causes when possible. Obviously, the first step of repair is a sincere apology. But is there anything else that can be done? In particular, what does the other person need to feel safe and respected? How can the harm be repaired to the fullest extent possible?

Reintegration - This is about what happens after the restorative process meeting. Each party must make good on any repair discussed. You have talked the talk, now you must walk the walk. This involves acceptance by all parties involved otherwise you may never move forward.

Another important part of reintegration is "meeting the person in front of you." That means that moving forward, you are seeing the person in front of you for who they are in that moment. You are not seeing them through the lens of past conflict. This is important because if we get stuck in previous conceptualizations of the person in front of us, we can never recognize their growth or change (and vice-versa).

Sometimes restorative processes work very well, other times not so much. You can only control your contribution to the process. However, if you follow the five R's and give each one its due, you are likely to have a meaningful inter-action and achieve some real repair of your relationships. Even if others are not sincere participants in the process, your sincerity and maturity will shine through in the eyes of the powers that be. This is critically important if you are under some kind of PIP or monitoring.

You can also see why we saved this chapter until the end. A great deal of introspection as well as skill building often needs to occur before a restorative process can be fruitful. Insight into our own stories about the incident in question, deep listening skills, and an understanding of how boundaries are violated are all necessary for a successful outcome.

CHAPTER ELEVEN

Job Crafting

Towards a workable future

If you have come this far, I want to commend you! Engaging in critical self-appraisal regarding your speech and behavior is not easy. It requires both willingness and vulnerability. In return for that hard work, I hope you have gained insight, knowledge, and practical skills.

Now it would be possible to end the book here. The specific problem areas reviewed to this point represent the bulk of what I see as an executive coach and advocate for physicians. Being able to see these pitfalls, and having a skill-set for navigating them, can go a long way towards bullet-proofing your career. If you do nothing more than master the material up to this point, you will have done yourself a great service.

However, I think there is benefit to spending a few moments zooming out and taking a 30,000 foot view as well. Interpersonal friction does not occur in a vacuum. Rather, it occurs in the context of our professional and personal lives as a whole. If our incredible hard work is not translating into a sense of fulfillment at the end of the day, or if we are unable to honor the other things in life that are important, then all of the pitfalls we have explored are more likely to occur.

As we have touched upon already, less than ideal behaviors often result from the neurocognitive impact of stress. If we have a chronic, high level of dissatisfaction and stress in our work or home lives, that is going to fuel poor communication, boundary issues, and disruptive behavior. We can master the ideas and skills discussed in the preceding individual chapters all we want, but if things aren't all right at a macro-level we are effectively handicapping ourselves.

Thus in my work with thousands of physicians, I have found that it is often not enough to just get granular and identify the individual areas of challenge. Rather, a holistic view is also necessary. That is what these final two chapters will focus on. In this chapter we will look at our work overall, and use a model to help us understand how we get stuck and how we thrive professionally. In the next chapter, we will assess our lives outside of work to do the same.

The Competency-Joy model of work

A simple but extremely effective for tool for understanding why our works feels the way it does is the Competency-Joy model. To use this model we take every task we do at work and ask two questions:

1. Does this task bring me joy / excitement?
2. Am I good at this task?

Combined, these two questions create four possible outcomes for any given task, which can then be sorted into a 2x2 matrix with four quadrants:

- Quadrant I: Tasks that I really enjoy/excite me, but I am not (yet) good at
- Quadrant II: Tasks that I really enjoy/excite me, and that I am good at
- Quadrant III: Tasks that I really do NOT enjoy/do not excite me, but I am good at

- Quadrant IV: Tasks that I really do NOT enjoy/do not excite me, and I am also not good at

We can then quantify how much time we spend on each task, and use this to determine how full each quadrant is relative to each other (with all quadrants adding up to 100% of our professional effort in terms of time).

The four seasons of professional development

Using this simple model we can gain some profound insights. Let's start by thinking back to medical school and early residency. Chances are at that point you were very excited to learn medicine and get your hands on patients. There was a lot that you were looking forward to professionally. At the same time, you were not (yet) very good at any of it. You had a mountain of material to learn and skills to acquire.

At this point in time Quadrant I was very full for you. Quadrant II was relatively empty, as you had not yet mastered much. Quadrant III was also relatively empty for the same reasons. Last, given that you were a student and your sole task was to learn, there likely wasn't a lot being asked of you yet that would fill Quadrant IV.

Visually, your Competency-Joy matrix likely looked like this:

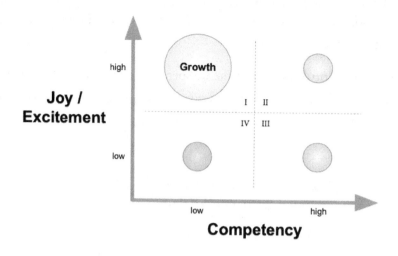

Diagram 2 - Early Training: The season of growth (Spring)

Another way to think about this is to use the four seasons as an analogy. When Quadrant I is relatively full as above, this is like being in Spring. We are embarking on a new chapter. There is a sense of adventure and commitment to the road ahead. We are putting in the hard work, preparing the soil and planting seeds so to speak. We are laying the foundation for a great harvest. It is early days and things are tenuous, but we can sense signs of life are about to emerge. We are in a growth phase, and this is why items in Quadrant I are referred to as *growth* tasks.

The growth of Spring, however, does not last forever. As our training progresses we do master our trade. We start to feel our competency. Things that we did not do well just a few years ago have become things that we are excited to do because now we do them well! We can bask a bit in our growing accomplishments. For many physicians, this starts to occur in later residency, fellowship, or the first years of being an attending.

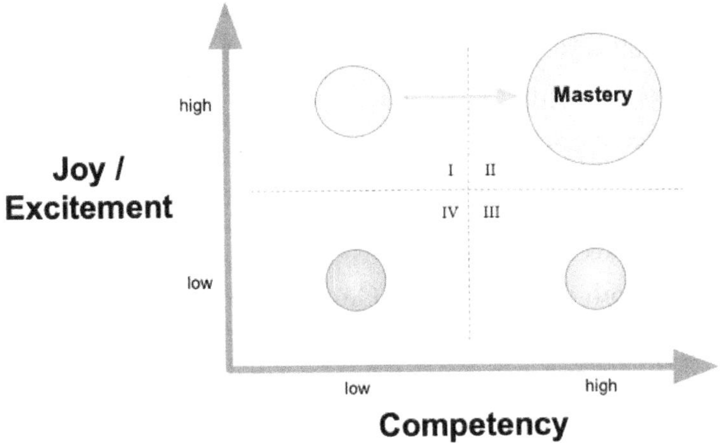
high
Mastery
Joy /
Excitement
I
II
IV
III
low
low
high
Competency

Diagram 3 - Late Training or Early Attending: The season of mastery (Summer)

Coming back to our "seasons" analogy, we can say we have entered Summer, the season of mastery. Everything is flourishing. There is a lushness and vitality. Graphically in our model this is represented by Quadrant II becoming more full as items migrate over from Quadrant I. At this point we have also likely realized that there are some tasks we have become good at but take little pleasure in (Quadrant III). Perhaps we are even noticing some thorns in our side being added to our plate, ie., tasks that we are not good at and have no desire to get good at (Quadrant IV). Nevertheless, Quadrant II mastery tasks and Quadrant I growth tasks still dominate our professional effort.

Now just as Spring does not last forever, neither does Summer. More and more mastery is obtained, but we start to notice that we savor this mastery less for some tasks. Some things we only dreamed of being able to achieve now seem rote. In our model, this is represented by Quadrant II tasks starting to migrate down to Quadrant III. We are still good at these things (in some cases very good - maybe even the best!), but they may not energize us as they once did.

In addition to things becoming rote, there are other reasons Quadrant III becomes more full with time. People see our competency and, thinking that we will do a good job, try to add things to our plate that are important *to them*. Being agreeable and conscientious, we take these things on and strive to do them well. This only prompts others to add even more tasks to our plate.

Pretty soon, for both of these reasons, Quadrant III becomes dominant. We find ourselves spending a lot of professional effort engaging in areas of mastery that just don't excite us as much anymore, or that represent *other people's* priorities and urgencies. We can do all of these things - in fact we do them well - which only masks the fact that much of what we are doing has become increasingly disconnected from our values and priorities. For this reason, Quadrant III activities are known as *disconnect* activities.

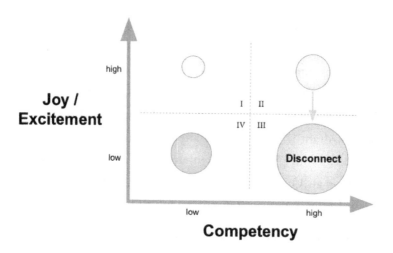

Diagram 4 - Sometime Post-Training: The season of disconnect (Autumn)

What is perhaps most interesting about these disconnect tasks is that they are actually the primary driver of burnout. People mistakenly assume that Quadrant IV activities are the most problematic for career satisfaction. In reality, its Quadrant III activities that erode at our soul.

After all, as highly intelligent problem-solvers we don't suffer Quadrant IV activities for long. We either get rid of them or we at least get good at them (shifting them to Quadrant III). In contrast, Quadrant III / disconnect activities are much more insidious. Having worked so hard at them for so long, it is difficult to acknowledge they bring us less joy and excitement than they once did. Also, because we do them well and often receive external praise for them, we are less likely to see Quadrant III activities as highly problematic. Thus there is a lot of inertia in our doing these activities. We are so busy "doing" that we often have no time to slow down and just "be" with these activities to see if they are really still in alignment with our joy and values.

And as Quadrant III momentum builds, our Joy-Competency matrix becomes bottom heavy. We can think of this as Autumn. Most of our plans have come to fruition and we have reaped what we have sowed. On one hand, it is easy to tell ourselves that we are in a good place. We have achieved so much and are recognized as someone who does things well. At the same time, we cant help but notice the vitality of summer is fading. Things have lost their luster. The joyful has become monotonous. We sense things have somehow peaked and we are now on a downward slide. We are competently doing more than ever, yet that is translating less and less into a sense of fulfillment at the end of the day.

This rate of progression of Spring to Summer to Autumn is highly variable for physicians. Some may find themselves in Autumn before even finishing their training, especially if fellowship was involved. For others, Autumn may not come until a decade or two as an attending. Regardless, this cycle *will* occur. Given a long enough time horizon, most of our professional activities slowly migrate from being growth opportunities to areas of mastery and ultimately to feeling rote (Quadrant I to II to III). They certainly won't all do this at once. Some tasks may even stay in Quadrant II for decades.

It is the trend over time that shifts the balance until the bottom half of the Competency-Joy matrix is relatively heavy. Eventually a tipping point will occur where things just feel different. Regardless of when this happens, we then face a choice. We can ignore the fading vitality around us, or we can get to work and change things.

Unfortunately, many physicians I have worked with have been doing the first option for years. They cling to what they have worked so hard for, convinced that it is still working for them. They also get stuck on the idea that once their training was over, everything was supposed to crystalize into some steady state where they could just enjoy the fruits of their labor in perpetuity as working attendings. Summer was supposed to be endless!

Thus the rude awakening that is Autumn often comes as a shock. Unwilling to face and question the growing sense of disconnect, physicians will often spend years convincing themselves that the feeling is temporary - that they are "just in a rut." They tell themselves, "Things will improve if I can just get to X (when my practice hires that new person, when COVID is over, when this merger is complete, when I get that grant, when I get promoted to Chief . . .).

But things don't get better when we don't face the disconnect. We eventually find ourselves in Winter. All vitality is gone. The world is less hospitable. It feels like getting through the day is more about survival than flourishing. There is a sense of loss of control, and often even grief for the Summer that has passed. This is true burnout.

Thus Winter occurs when we ignore what Autumn is telling us, but is there another way? Can we at least slow the progression of the seasons, or maybe even bypass Winter entirely and find an early Spring? The answer is yes. Through a combination of job crafting, identifying new growth opportunities, and changing our mindset towards certain aspects of our work, we can re-adjust the balance of our own Competency-Joy Matrix.

Perhaps most importantly, the balance does not need to be as top heavy as you might imagine. Research on physician well-being from the Mayo Clinic has shown that when physicians engage in activities that give them joy and excitement just 20% of the time, they halve their risk for burnout and their job satisfaction jumps dramatically. Of course more is better, but 20% appears to be a critical threshold.

Twenty percent is manageable! It is the equivalent of one workday out of five. It means that we can still have plenty of obligatory activities and thorns in our side and still manage to go home with a sense of fulfillment at the end of the day.

Finding twenty percent

So how do we intentionally re-balance our matrix? To do so, we first need to understand what our own matrix really looks like.

In my experience talking to countless physicians, I have noticed most know exactly what they do on a daily basis. If I ask them to account for their time down to 15 minute increments, they can. However, if I ask them to quantify how each activity *feels*, they have much more trouble. Most physicians can qualify their work satisfaction globally, but beyond that things get murky. This makes sense! After all, we are all so busy *doing* on a daily basis, we have no time to ask ourselves how each activity *feels*. We just know, overall, how we feel cumulatively at the end of the day.

So the first step in re-balancing our matrix is to get granular. To do this I have my clients document their daily activities in as much detail as possible down to 15 minute increments, and to reflect on how each block of time felt. Usually one to two weeks of this is more than enough to generate real insight. It often isn't until someone does this level of reflection that they are able to notice, for example, that it is not *all* patient care that is draining them, but rather a certain subset of cases that are coloring their entire experience. Or maybe through this exercise they realize just how different one clinical site feels versus another site that they also practice at. Or maybe they realize just how much they actually enjoy the QA/patient safety committee work that they do, or how much they despise it and how much time it actually takes away from other things. Or maybe they see that there is one person that is highly problematic and affecting other aspects of their work.

Regardless, once you have done this you can really understand what percentage of your professional effort is filing which quadrants, and most importantly, why. From this starting point, you can systematically address each quadrant.

Growing Quadrant I

Most of us love to learn and be challenged. It is why many of us went to medical school in the first place. Not surprisingly, when Quadrant I atrophies, so do we. Thus Quadrant I represents low hanging fruit in terms of reinvigorating our matrix.

The paradox, however, is that this often the last thing we want to do when we are burned out. When we are in Autumn or Winter, the idea of adding more challenges and more things to our plate is overwhelming. Our instinct is to withdraw, not to engage more. However, adding more to our plate may be just what the doctor ordered. In fact, at least two studies have shown that when physicians experience burnout, those who take on new activities reduce their burnout scores considerably more than those who do not.

The key is that you have to take on the *right* activities - meaning activities that truly excite you! If you take on other peoples' priorities and things that they are excited about, you are only adding to Quadrant III. So where is your growth edge? A great way to determine this is using an exercise called "The Three Questions."

Now before you do this exercise, a few instructions. First, you need a timer and you need to limit your responses to 90 seconds for each question. You could easily spend an hour on each question, but the goal is to see what comes up first. Also, keep writing for the 90 seconds in a stream-of-consciousness fashion, not complete sentences. Last, don't focus on being practical or try to talk yourself out of something due to perceived limitations. This is a wish list, so give yourself permission to imagine that anything is possible.

So with those instructions in mind, spend 90 seconds each writing out answers to the following three questions:

- In the next year or two, what do you want to experience/have happen professionally?
- In the next year or two, what new skills or learning do you want to acquire?
- In the next year or two, how do you want to contribute to your organization or your field?

If it's been a long time since you've asked yourself such questions, it may be very hard to come up with answers. That is ok! It just means the exercise is all that more important to you at this point in your life. If you need to do this a few times over a couple of weeks, then do so.

Once you have a list, it's time to get to work. What would it take to make some of these things happen? Even if something seems like a massive undertaking, what is the next natural small step you could take this week or this month in that direction? What mini-experiments can you craft to dip your toes into a potential area of interest? With each step, you will be refilling Quadrant I. This intrinsically feels good (assuming you are taking on new things that are really in line with *your* passions and values). Also, Quadrant I is the fuel for Quadrant II growth.

Only you can find growth opportunities that are meaningful to you. The following are some examples of changes that physicians I have worked with have made a result of their Three Question Exercise:

- Shifting the types of cases they focus on
- Learning a new procedure or tool
- Spending more time in a preferred clinical setting (in-patient, out-patient, different clinical site, etc)
- Taking on a leadership/committee role in an area of true interest (and not because it would look good on their CV or their department chair "volun-told" them to do it)
- Leaving private practice for academics so as to teach more, or vice-versa
- Taking on a meaningful research or administrative project, or getting rid of research or administrative projects that do not excite them
- Reducing to part time to take on a non-clinical opportunity that uses their MD/DO
- Finding a new employer where growth opportunities in their area of interest are greater
- Leaving medicine because there are other skills and talents they wish to grow
- Developing leadership, conflict resolution, or communication skills
- Pursuing another degree or fellowship because of a deep personal interest (and not for the "merit badge" letters at the end of their name)

Regardless of what growth opportunities you craft for yourself, the important things is that you *do* craft new growth opportunities. This is something no one ever tells us in our training, and it can be a painful truth to learn: growth is not a phase of our career development. Rather, it is necessary to stoke the fires of growth in perpetuity. The challenge, however, is that this is a habit we fall out of early on. After all, once we decided to become physicians, the medical education system filled Quadrant I for us for many years. Then one day we were done with our training, and no one told us it was now our turn to keep adding fuel to the fire.

Growing Quadrant II

As made clear by the Competency-Joy model, Quadrant II is fueled by Quadrant I. If we don't have a strong growth edge, there are no growth tasks that can mature into activities that we enjoy *and* are competent at. Thus in one respect we can't grow Quadrant II directly, we can only feed Quadrant I. This makes Quadrant I work all the more important to focus on.

That said, however, there are ways we can strengthen our experience of Quadrant II by making it *feel* bigger. One thing I have noticed about our culture as physicians is that we do not allow ourselves to savor our achievements. We may accomplish something very significant, but as soon as we do, we discount our newfound success and turn our focus to the next desired line item on our CV.

It also doesn't help that we are surrounded by people who do the same things that we do on a daily basis. For example, you may do tremendously meaningful work as an oncologist. Everyone you work with is also an oncologist doing the same. *Relatively* it seems less special. As such, the uniqueness and importance of what you contribute to the world can get lost. This is a problem that is not limited to medicine, but actually pervades most high-performing professions.

This is so problematic because it means that we do not recognize Quadrant II activities for what they are. We discount our own mastery and fail to savor the joy and excitement because we are taught in medicine that that is somehow selfish. Doing so will also make us somehow become complacent and lose our edge. The result is that Quadrant II never *feels* full because we never allow ourselves to savor it. Rather, some Quadrant II activities get relegated quickly to Quadrant III in our minds even though they shouldn't.

Fortunately, there is great neuroscience research that demonstrates that we can counteract this. The bulk of these tools fall into two categories - *values* and *gratitude*.

Values exercises are so fruitful that they are now consistently one of the first things I do with a physician regardless of the reason I am working with them. To start, I begin by defining values, because they may not be what you think. *Family, work, health* - these things are not values. You may value them, but they are not what we mean when we talk about values. Rather, they are simply who and what are important to you.

Values, by contrast, are verbs and adverbs. They are the qualities of behavior that you bring to who and what is valuable to you. You may love your family, but how do you want to be when you engage with them? Is it more important to you to bring a sense of adventure, or authenticity? Fairness or independence? Tolerance or honesty? Now of course all of these values may be good things, but each of us has 5 or 6 core values that we tend to embrace over all others.

So what are your core values? A very helpful exercise in this regard can be found in Appendix Three. I encourage you to take 15 minutes and complete it now to generate your 5 or 6 core values. Assuming you were honest with yourself, these 5 or 6 values should feel like the true you. They are likely life-long qualities that you have embraced. Looking back at the times you thrived in life, it was likely due to you living these values well. Similarly, times you languished were likely times you were less able to bring these values to bear on your day-to-day activities.

With this in mind, how are you living your values now in your professional capacity? Go through each value one by one, and think of all the tasks you do. Make a list of all the ways your values manifest in what you do whether big or small. The power in creating this list is that it reminds us of where we feel connected to our work on a daily basis, and so we feel the joy of Quadrant II activities more. Also, it is not uncommon that when you start to view tasks through a sense of values and purpose, some can migrate back from Quadrant III to Quadrant II.

Similar to values, the research is overwhelming that gratitude exercises can have a similar effect on well being, and further augment the impact of connecting with values. By gratitude, we are referring to any structure or exercise that helps you savor that which is good. There are many exercises and apps out there that can be helpful, but my favorite involves asking a few simple questions once a week. The idea is to reflect on the prior week, and answer each question by journaling for a minute or so on each. Also, it does not matter how small the moment or action was, it is more important to generate an answer:

- Where is one time you made a difference?
- What is one moment of connection that you experienced with a patient or colleague?
- Where is one instance where you were able to live your values in your work?
- What is one moment you felt connected to your sense of purpose?
- What is one moment when you laughed?

Studies have shown that for physicians and other providers, doing an exercise like this once a week can have a notable impact on burnout and job satisfaction. These types of exercise are not about being "Pollyanna-ish" and ignoring the negative. Rather, they help overcome the strong negative bias we all have, especially under chronic stress. They allow for a more balanced and realistic assessment of our day-to-day experience.

Connectivity with values and gratitude can help us savor those things that are actually in Quadrant II, making it feel bigger. Also, when we view Quadrant

III tasks through our values they can sometimes take on new meaning, moving them at least partially back towards Quadrant II.

Minimizing Quadrant III

Thus far our focus has been to make Quadrants I and II bigger. At the same time, we can work on making Quadrants III and IV smaller, because it is the ratio that matters.

Regarding Quadrant III, we will never be able to eliminate all the activities in it. There will be things we are good at that are required for our job that we just don't enjoy. They are the price we pay, so to speak, to be able to do the good stuff. However, most people find that if they are being truly honest with themselves, much of what is in Quadrant III is often the result of weak boundaries.

Boundaries are simply what we say "yes" and "no" to, and physicians are terrible at saying "no." Instead, our lives are filled with "should" and "ought."

- I ought to do this because it would look good on my CV.
- I should say yes to this request to minimize friction.
- I should keep doing this specific activity because I am good at it.
- I ought to be grateful for my job security / income (and therefore have no right to complain or make changes)

The result of all of this "should-ing" all over ourselves is we often allow other people to put their priorities and needs on our plate, and we don't push back. We also keep doing certain activities because of inertia - people see us as the person who does X, and we can't let them down! Ultimately, we feel resent- ment or overwhelm, which are the hallmarks of weak boundaries.

Fortunately, this is mitigable with stronger boundaries. So I challenge you, where can you start saying "no" more? Here are a few reflection questions to stimulate your thinking:

- Where is one place you should not have said "yes" to something or someone in the last month?
- Where are you spending a lot of time and energy on someone else's priority?
- Where is one place you could be saying "no" even more than you already are?
- Where are you afraid you might disappoint someone else if you acted differently?
- What is one activity where your heart just isn't in it anymore?
- Where do you see someone else saying "no" that you wish you could do the same?

These are tough questions. The answers, however, are key for identifying where you can take action. Start small and give yourself self-compassion, as this is some of the hardest job-crafting that you can do. Boundaries are emotional for you and for others, so this is likely to be friction filled. Also, as physicians, boundaries have been trained out of us. We have been taught that boundaries are self-indulgent, so don't be surprised if you feel guilt.

Given the lack of boundaries that is part and parcel of our medical training, and given that many of us were conscientious people even prior to medical school, many of us likely need a *lot* of work regarding boundaries. That work may take years. It is, however, critical to do. Just as you don't become a full-fledged adult until you develop strong, healthy boundaries with your parents and siblings, you don't become a fully developed professional until you develop strong, healthy boundaries with your work.

So if you find yourself challenged by this material, I strongly encourage you to tap other resources. I often recommend the works of Nedra Glover Tawwab, MSW, LCSW and Sarri Gilman, MA, MFT as starting points. There are also a lot of great resources online. As you read these resources, you will notice much of the discussion of boundaries is in the context of relationships, and that is ok. Let's be honest, medicine is probably one of the biggest and most intimate relationships you have. When you conceptualize your work in that way, as a living relationship, you will see the same problems and strategies that apply to your spouse or parents are also applicable to your job and employer.

Minimizing Quadrant IV

Last we come to Quadrant IV - full of things we don't enjoy and are not good at. These tend to be more technical and menial tasks. Nonetheless, it should be noted that activities can exist in Quadrant IV for the same reasons they exist in Quadrant III - boundaries. So first ask yourself all of the questions above. What can you say no to? Are there boundaries that need to be expressed? Remember, the more balls you appear able to juggle, the more balls people will give you to juggle.

Now if you can't outright say no to these tasks on your plate, then the next best strategy is to see what you can delegate. Are you making full use of other providers and support staff, or are you micromanaging and reluctant to trust others to do the work? To function at the highest level of our licensure we often have to trust and empower others around us to do the same.

Delegation also relates to technology. Using pre-written templates or alternative means of documentation (like voice recognition or scribes) are forms of delegating. Are you truly masterful at your EHR, or did you just learn enough to get by and finish your notes? It is worth asking because EHR systems often have incredible tools for managing workflow that we are never taught. By putting in the time to become a "super-user," or finding someone who is, you can often find ways to leverage the technology and offload some of your effort onto the tech itself.

Lastly, if you cant stop doing it, and you can't delegate it, you can at least get better at a given task. If it is a choice between being unexcited and unskilled at something, versus unexcited but at least skilled at that thing, choose the latter as it is more efficient. So ask yourself, what skills or knowledge have you been avoiding that could probably improve the quality of your day if you just bit the bullet and learned them? EHR? Documentation and coding compliance? Conflict resolution skills? Leadership and management strategies? It is extremely hard to put time and effort into becoming good at something we have no interest in, especially when we are already overwhelmed. However, if we truly can't escape doing something, we can at least minimize our own suffering.

Crafting a better tomorrow

The Competency-Joy Model, and all of the strategies above, are really in service of the idea of job crafting. How can we change our activities and interactions so that we are more fulfilled at the end of the day? Where can we re-invigorate our growth edge? How can we connect with and savor our mastery more? What boundaries do we need to honor? What can we take off of our plates or at least make more palatable?

When we ask these questions, we have the opportunity to optimize our current work environment. Unfortunately, sometimes that may not be enough. Sometimes the work of job crafting reveals that we simply cannot remain in our current role or at our current organization. Or sometimes we try to job craft in a few different organizations over time, only to discover that the problem is medicine itself, and it is time to pursue non-clinical jobs. Regardless, the only way to know what we need is to have a step-wise approach, which is what the Competency-Joy Model gives us.

CHAPTER TWELVE

The Wheel of Life

Everything else that matters!

The previous chapter focused on how to systematically analyze and improve our work experience by taking the 30,000 foot view. In this chapter, we take the 50,000 foot view and use a similar model to see how all of the pieces of our lives fit together.

This is so important because, in my experience, I have found that it is not uncommon for stressors and misalignments outside of work to be the primary drivers of chronic stress and burnout *at work*. I can't tell you how many times a physician has said to me that they are burned out and ready to leave medicine, and yet when we get granular, it becomes clear that for them the practice of medicine is actually intrinsically enjoyable. Rather, it's the friction or neglect in other major areas of their life that is the problem. These types of issues can be just as detrimental to our well-being as a lack of fulfillment in the work itself, and can ultimately fuel the incidents that lead many people to read this book!

The Wheel of Life

Our lives have many areas of importance: work, health, relationships, and fun/leisure are the big four, but there are many others including personal development, spirituality/religion, or parenting.

Unfortunately, what happens for many high-performing professionals is that all of these are deferred in the name of professional development when we are young adults. In our twenties and even thirties our professional growth was our primary focus. All of the other things had to be wedged in along the margins. But that was ok, because our lives were also relatively simple. No one was relying on us - we could do our own thing! We may have had a significant other but that was likely the only major relationship we had to navigate. Most of us could count on being healthy. Similarly our parents were likely also relatively healthy. Yes, work took a tremendous amount of time, but the time that was left was ours to use as we pleased.

But then we grew up. Relationships, especially with significant others, became more complex and enmeshed. Perhaps we had children and were now responsible for a whole lot more than ourselves. Our health could no longer be taken for granted. Some us developed chronic medical conditions, and all of us became more acutely aware of the limitations of how hard we could push ourselves. Our parents or other older loved ones may have developed greater needs as well. Finances became far more complicated.

Here lies the problem. Having prioritized our work for so long, and having not had to think as much about these other things, many of us suddenly turn around one day and realize how out of balance things are. Unintentionally, we realize we have engaged in a lot of blind neglect.

This is where the Wheel of Life exercise comes in - to ask some hard questions and to create a blueprint for change. The actual exercise is in Appendix Four for your reference as we walk through the following steps.

First, please rank the 8 areas of life in order of importance. Of course, almost every area mentioned is important, but I am asking you to take a stand. No ties, no half points - just a numerical ranking 1 through 8.

Once you have done that, then follow the remainder of the instructions in Appendix Four. Ultimately, you will create a wheel which serves as a visual representation of your satisfaction in each of these areas over the last few months.

Now looking at your completed wheel, what is your initial reaction or impression? Take a few moments to write down your thoughts.

Next, imagine that this is the wheel upon which you "roll through life." Is the ride smooth, or do you jolt along as unbalanced areas each come to the fore? Again, take a few moments to write your answers.

Now keeping with the metaphor of the wheel, I want you to imagine that each of our wheels turns at a constant rate throughout our lives. Despite the constant rate, our wheel tends to change shape and size. At some points in our life the wheel may be very large (many areas rated highly). When that is the case we metaphorically cover more distance with each turn - which results in greater vitality and meaning. When the diameter is very small overall, it can feel like we are spinning our wheels but covering little ground, and so we feel stuck. Given this, how do you feel about how your wheel is working for you?

Lastly, take a few moments to look at the areas you rated the highest in satisfaction. What are you doing in those areas that leads to vitality? What values are being honored in those areas that might account for the higher score? What strengths and qualities are bringing to these areas? Similarly, look at the areas you rated lowest in satisfaction. What values are you less connected to that might account for the lower score?

Working the wheel

Now that you have explored your own wheel, it is time to get to work! I encourage professionals that I work with to start by looking at the areas of greatest mismatch. For example, perhaps you rated your satisfaction with Spirituality/Religion a 3 out of 10. That is a low number, but it also matters how highly you rated that area in terms of *importance*. If you ranked it #8 (lowest in importance of all of the areas), that is very different than if you ranked it #2. Similarly, perhaps you rated an area 7 out of 10 in terms of satisfaction, but also ranked that area #1 in terms of overall importance. In that case, perhaps a 7/10 feels like a real gap between where you are and where you want to be. So where is your biggest mismatch in terms of relatively low satisfaction but relatively high importance? That is likely the area where you will get the biggest bang for your buck in terms of effort.

Having identified that area, it's time to come up with short-, medium-, and long-term goals for change. What would it take for you to rank that area just 0.5 points higher in terms of satisfaction a month or two from now? Similarly, what would it take for you to rank that area two points higher a year or two from now? Be specific in terms of how you would quantify this. What would really have to happen or change? What would others notice was different about you?

Take some time to really flesh this out and write it down. What are realistic goals in the next month or two, next three to nine months, and next one to two years? Also, this is a place where the values exercise from the previous chapter can be extremely helpful. If you are having trouble conceptualizing what changes might be helpful, you can look at each core value and how you might express it more in the area in question.

As you do this for yourself, it can also help to see an example of how this has helped others:

Samantha was a young attending in private-practice anesthesiology. Over the last 6-12 months, she had noticed a change in how work felt. There was a sense of just "working for a paycheck" and she felt less invested in her patients and colleagues. Nothing bad had happened yet, but she was vulnerable to a patient complaint or interpersonal misunderstanding.

A few close friends and colleagues had noticed this as well, and one recommended that she work with a physician career coach. Starting with the Competency-Joy Matrix, she realized that work itself was actually better than she thought. She had areas of growth that she was looking forward to, she did still enjoy many of her clinical tasks, and she had reasonable boundaries (in fact, private-practice anesthesiology was a direct expression of those boundaries).

Next, she did the Wheel of Life. Her first big insight came when she saw her wheel, which was full with the glaring exception of finances, which she rated 3 out of 10. As she started to explore this with her coach, she explained how she had grown up quite poor with a tremendous amount of financial instability. As long as she could remember, she had told herself that this would not happen to her as an adult. In fact, some of the appeal of medicine in the first place was the six-figure income and exceptional job security. Not surprisingly, this was also reflected in her Core Values Exercise where security, independence, stability, and competence emerged as her most tightly-held values.

But when she looked at her current life, there was a significant misalignment. Once that first paycheck as an attending came, she made up for lost time and spent very freely. After all, she deserved it! She had about $15,000 in credit card debt, a very expensive car, and a ritzy downtown apartment with high monthly payments. While she liked these things, she simultaneously worried about the future she hoped to have when she had a family of her own.

Also, given her background, she had to take on a large amount of debt to make it through college and medical school. She was able to make her required payments on this debt month to month, but at the same time she had to admit it terrified her and she had very little knowledge of the intricacies of managing that kind of debt.

This was her "ah-ha" moment. She realized her resentment towards her work was not intrinsic to the work itself. Rather, she resented that despite how hard she had worked, she did not have the life or stability that she imagined. Despite now making literally 10 times her family's income when she was a child, she did not feel safe or independent because she needed every dollar of her paycheck and felt trapped. Yes, she had money finally, but she lacked the competence to make it work for her.

So with this insight, she came up with a longitudinal plan. She worked for a bit with a therapist because there was clearly unresolved trauma from her upbringing. She pursued education around finances through courses and personal finance books. These initial steps allowed her to engage with her debt. The initial math shocked her and there were times she wanted to crawl back in the hole, but with a little self-compassion and accountability from her coach she was able to create a comprehensive plan.

Within a year she had eliminated her credit card debt, refinanced her educational debt, and was more aggressively paying it down. Within two years she had moved, bought a cheaper car, and was more intentional about her spending. She came to value experiences over material items. Most importantly, she came to understand that her ignoring her debt and spending freely made her feel powerful over money in the moment, but undermined her values and goals in the long term.

And as she did all of this, work became enjoyable again. Reducing the stressor outside of work had a tremendous impact on her experience of work.

Now not everyone of us will have a glaring area that needs attention like Samantha above. However, every one of us can benefit from attending to our Wheel of Life. Our professional endeavors do not exist in a vacuum. We do not have separate emotional, cognitive, and spiritual gas tanks for work versus for the rest of life. If the pieces are not working together and somewhat in balance, then none of it works well. This erodes our professional well-being, setting us up for professional friction.

In contrast, a smooth, full wheel can propel us forward. When all of the pieces are reasonably in balance they can work together to buffer the inevitable rough spots we will encounter in one area or another. Most importantly, we will enjoy the ride!

AFTERWORD

I want to commend you! The work in this book is not easy. The circumstances leading you to read this book in the first place may also not have been easy. Nonetheless, I hope you found it valuable.

Not everyone will need everything in this book. But most physicians will need a lot of what is in this book. I imagine some areas were eye opening, while others felt like common sense. If what you read simply reinforced things you are already doing, then that is great. If what you read revealed a major area of challenge, that is great too. Either way, you should have a much stronger skill set for navigating the modern healthcare work environment.

Remember that every story in this book is real. Names and details have been changed, but the events occurred to one of your peers and can occur to you too. Learn from these examples so that you don't have to experience them in the future.

So use this book, work with a coach, educate yourself. Do whatever it takes to bulletproof your career. You have worked too hard to lose the ability to practice clinical medicine the way you want to. In the process, you might also find that your days are much more enjoyable! For all of the practical talk about safeguarding your career, the ideas and skills in this book are just as much about improving *your* day-to-day experience of your work. Because not only do you deserve to be able to continue working, you deserve to actually enjoy it too!

Ryan Bayley, MD is an executive coach and physician advocate who has worked with thousands of clinicians to optimize their careers and happiness. To that end, he is the founder of Bayley Coaching Solutions, a physician-focused executive coaching and consulting firm. His group works with multiple states' medical boards and physician health programs, as well as individual healthcare organizations. In addition to his coaching and consulting work, he is a nationally recognized speaker and author, as well as a consultant to large healthcare organizations.

Dr. Bayley completed his undergraduate at Harvard, and subsequently attended Vanderbilt Medical School. He completed his residency in emergency medicine at Columbia and Cornell Universities (New York-Presbyterian) and his EMS fellowship with the Fire Department of New York. In addition to his executive coaching and consulting, he still practices emergency medicine and serves as an emergency medical services director for 911 systems. He also currently holds an associate adjunct position at Duke University Medical Center, where he leads courses on physician well-being and career design.

If you or your organization are interested in keynotes, workshops, or individual / group coaching do not hesitate to reach out!

www.solvingcareers.com

The "My Narrative" Exercise

This is a narrative writing exercise designed to further explore the event(s) that led to reading this book. If such an event does not apply to you, you can use this exercise to explore any challenging and friction-filled interpersonal situation in your professional work.

Once you have an event in mind, the first step is to write out what happened. Imagine that you are writing this in a letter to your closest friend and most trusted confidant. You can be completely open and honest. Take about 15-20 minutes and really tell your story. Who did what? How did things come to be? What was your role? What where others' roles? What motives did everyone have? What was going on behind the scenes? It is necessary that you actually write this out and not just reflect on it. Take the time to do that now.

Now you have your story written down. It may look something like the following example that we will use to work through this exercise:

> "... Late on Friday I was waiting patiently to start my last case. The OR manager came and found me in the hallway. She claimed that I did not have my consent form in the chart and therefore the case could not start. She does this whenever her staff is overwhelmed with room turnover so that it doesn't look like the problem is with her team. I told her I was certain it was in the chart - I knew for a fact I had put it there about an

hour ago! She has such an ego and doesn't like pushback, so not surprisingly she started getting all bent out of shape because I was calling her bluff. I stepped between her and the two medical students I was with to indicate that I did not think this was professional. I pointed to her office and said we should go talk, and when she turned I put my hand on her shoulder to walk with her there . . . "

Regardless of the specifics of your story, it is now time to separate objective fact from interpretation. Go through and put a line through everything that was your opinion or your mind-reading of other peoples' thoughts and intent. Cross out things that only you could have known. Also, replace any reference to something that you or something others said with the specific quote, rather than paraphrasing. Last, when you find something that was interpretation, you can also feel free to re-word it to reflect only what was objectively observable.

Imagine a film crew was following you around doing a documentary. What would the camera have seen and heard? Cameras don't know thoughts or intent. They don't have memories or associations with past events. They are objective and precise.

Returning to our example above, this next step could look like this:

" . . . Late on Friday I was waiting ~~patiently~~ to start my last case. The OR manager came and found me in the hallway. ~~She claimed that I did not have my consent form in the chart and therefore the case could not start.~~ She said, "The CRNA cannot find your consent and we need it to start the case." ~~She does this whenever her staff is overwhelmed with room turnover so that it doesn't look like the problem is with her team. I told her I was certain it was in the chart—I knew for a fact I had put it there about an hour ago!~~ I said, "This is ridiculous, it is in there, look again." ~~She has such an ego and doesn't like pushback, so not surprisingly she started getting all bent out of shape because I was calling her bluff.~~

***She raised her voice.** I stepped between her and the two medical students I was with ~~to indicate that I did not think this was professional.~~ I pointed to her office and said ~~we should go talk,~~ "**Let's get in there.**" and when she turned I put my hand on her shoulder ~~to walk with her there~~ . . . "*

Now take a moment to look at your edited letter. How much is crossed out? Likely a lot. It is not uncommon for 75% of what you originally wrote to be crossed out or rephrased. Part of this exercise is to demonstrate just how much any narrative contains subjective interpretation in the form of assumptions regarding others' speech and motives, mind reading, and assuming others are privy to the same information that we have and are coming to the same conclusions based on that information.

As the final step in this exercise, take a moment to imagine how the skeleton of events that you have created could be filled back in with someone else's interpretation. For example, the event that you wrote about may have resulted in you being accused of poor communication, boundary issues, or disruptive behavior. How could you re-write the narrative (substituting others' interpretations for your own) in order to come to *their* conclusion?

To be clear, this is not about being right or wrong. You do not have to agree with their interpretation. The goal is simply to see that another interpretation is possible. This will require a little imagination and perspective taking. Regardless, it is important to see how multiple narratives can be derived from one common set of events.

Control Spectrum Worksheet

Take a moment to recall a challenging or friction-filled moment (really any moment of distress where unwanted thoughts, feelings, associations showed up). In a sentence or two, what was the situation? What were the core thoughts, feelings, associations, or memories showing up in this moment?

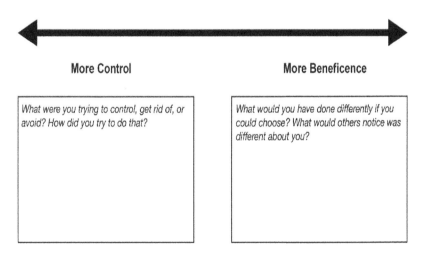

More Control

What were you trying to control, get rid of, or avoid? How did you try to do that?

More Beneficence

What would you have done differently if you could choose? What would others notice was different about you?

1. Place on X on the line above to indicate were you fell on the spectrum during this moment.

2. What were the costs of focusing on control?

3. What alternative behaviors would indicate that you were moving towards more beneficence and meaning?

4. Who or what can help you do more of that?

Adapted from the work of Strosahl, et. al. Brief Interventions for Radical Change, 2012

Values Sort

When you ask someone what they value, they will often say things like "family," "health," or "my work." In coaching, however, we don't consider these values; rather, they are important life areas.

Values, by contrast, refer to how you want to be when living each of these life areas. When you are being your best self in regards to health, for example, what does that look like?

In other words, <u>values are qualities of behavior</u> that we bring to the important areas of our life. Values are also not goals - they are not about what you want to get or achieve. Instead, they are about how you want to behave or act on an ongoing basis.

Most people will find the values on the following list to be "good things." However, when push comes to shove, most of us have five or six core values that we would like to live above all others. This exercise is about defining those and taking a stand!

So read through the list below and write a letter next to each value: V = Very Important, Q = Quite Important, and N = Not So Important. Be discerning, especially with the "Very Important" category. On this first pass you want to limit the number of values you identify as very important to about 10 or 15 at most. After all, if you rank most values as "Very Important" then that means that none of them are truly important!

Also, do this exercise as quickly as possible. Go with your gut instinct - don't overthink. You will have an opportunity to make changes later but for now it is about making a quick first pass.

1. Acceptance: to be open to and accepting of myself, others, life etc

2. Accuracy: to be accurate in my opinions and beliefs

3. Achievement: to have important accomplishments

4. Adventure: to be adventurous; to actively seek, create, or explore novel or stimulating experiences

5. Assertiveness: to respectfully stand up for my rights and request what I want

6. Authenticity: to be authentic, genuine, real; to be true to myself

7. Authority: to be in charge and responsible for others

8. Autonomy: to be self-determined and independent

9. Beauty: to appreciate, create, nurture or cultivate beauty in myself, others, the environment etc

10. Caring: to be caring towards myself, others, the environment etc

11. Challenge: to keep challenging myself to grow, learn, improve

12. Change: to have a life full of change and variety

13. Comfort: to have a pleasant and comfortable life

14. Compassion: to act with kindness towards those who are suffering

15. Connection: to engage fully in whatever I am doing, and be fully present with other

16. Contribution: to contribute, help, assist, or make a positive difference to myself or others

17. Conformity: to be respectful and obedient of rules and obligations

18. Cooperation: to be cooperative and collaborative with others

19. Courage: to be courageous or brave; to persist in the face of fear, threat, or difficulty

20. Courtesy: to be considerate and polite towards others

21. Creativity: to be creative or innovative

22. Curiosity: to be curious, open-minded and interested; to explore and discover

23. Dependability: to be reliable and trustworthy

24. Duty: to carry out my duties and obligations

25. Ecology: to live in harmony with the environment

26. Encouragement: to encourage and reward behavior that I value in myself or others

27. Equality: to treat others as equal to myself, and vice-versa

28. Excitement: to seek, create and engage in activities that are exciting, stimulating or thrilling

29. Faithfulness: to be loyal and true in relationships

30. Fairness: to be fair to myself or others

31. Fitness: to maintain or improve my fitness; to look after my physical and mental health and wellbeing

32. Flexibility: to adjust and adapt readily to changing circumstances

33. Freedom: to live freely; to choose how I live and behave, or help others do likewise

34. Friendliness: to be friendly, companionable, or agreeable towards others

35. Forgiveness: to be forgiving towards myself or others

36. Fun: to be fun-loving; to seek, create, and engage in fun-filled activities

37. Generosity: to be generous, sharing and giving, to myself or others

38. Genuineness: to act in a manner that is true to who I am

39. Gratitude: to be grateful for and appreciative of the positive aspects of myself, others, and life

40. Growth: to keep changing and growing

41. Helpfulness: to be helpful to others

42. Honesty: to be honest, truthful, and sincere with myself and others

43. Hope: to maintain a positive and optimistic outlook

44. Humility: to be humble or modest; to let my achievements speak for themselves

45. Humor: to see and appreciate the humorous side of life

46. Independence: to be self-supportive, and choose my own way of doing things

47. Industry: to be industrious, hard-working, dedicated

48. Intimacy: to open up, reveal, and share myself -- emotionally or physically – in my close personal relationships

49. Justice: to uphold justice and fairness

50. Kindness: to be kind, compassionate, considerate, nurturing or caring towards myself or others

51. Knowledge: to learn and contribute valuable knowledge

52. Leisure: to take to relax and enjoy

53. Love: to act lovingly or affectionately towards myself or others

54. Mastery: to be competent in my everyday activities

55. Mindfulness: to be conscious of, open to, and curious about my here-and-now experience

56. Moderation: to avoid excess and find a middle ground

57. Non-conformity: to question and challenge authority and norms

58. Nurturance: to take care of and nurture others

59. Order: to be orderly and organized

60. Open-mindedness: to think things through, see things from other's points of view, and weigh evidence fairly

61. Passion: to have deep feelings about ideas, activity, or people

62. Patience: to wait calmly for what I want

63. Persistence: to continue resolutely, despite problems or difficulties.

64. Pleasure: to create and give pleasure to myself or others

65. Power: to strongly influence or wield authority over others, e.g. taking charge, leading, organizing

66. Rationality: to be guided by reason and logic

67. Realism: to seek and act realistically and practically

68. Reciprocity: to build relationships in which there is a fair balance of giving and taking

69. Respect: to be respectful towards myself or others; to be polite, considerate and show positive regard

70. Responsibility: to be responsible and accountable for my actions

71. Risk: to take risks and chances

72. Romance: to be romantic; to display and express love or strong affection

73. Safety: to secure, protect, or ensure safety of myself or others

74. Self-acceptance: to accept myself as I am

75. Self-awareness: to be aware of my own thoughts, feelings, and actions

76. Self-care: to look after my health and wellbeing, and get my needs met

77. Self-control: to act in accordance with my own ideals and be disciplined

78. Self-development: to keep growing, advancing or improving in knowledge, skills, character, or life experience.

79. Sensuality: to create, explore, and enjoy experiences that stimulate the five senses

80. Service: to be of service to others

81. Sexuality: to explore or express my sexuality

82. Simplicity: to live life simply, with minimal needs

83. Skillfulness: to continually practice and improve my skills, and apply myself fully when using them

84. Solitude: to have time and space apart

85. Spirituality: to connect with things bigger than myself

86. Stability: to have life that stays daily constant

87. Supportiveness: to be supportive, helpful, encouraging, and available to myself or others

88. Tolerance: to accept and respect those different from me

89. Trust: to be trustworthy; to be loyal, faithful, sincere, and reliable

90. Virtue: to live a morally pure and excellent life

91. Insert your own unlisted value(s) here:

Once you've marked each value as V, Q, N (Very, Quite, or Not So Important), go through all the Vs and write them on a blank piece of paper. You will likely notice that some are very similar (i.e., getting at the same core concept based on your interpretation of the words). If so, group those together and choose the one that is most representative of what you value and cross out the other similar ones.

If there are still more than six Very Important values / values clusters after this step, select out the top five or six that are <u>most</u> important to you.

Sometimes when combining your Very Important values you find yourself with less than five. If that is the case, take a moment to look at your Quite Important list. Are there any values / values clusters that jump out that you would promote to your Very Important list?

Ultimately, we are trying to get at five to six core values. Finally, write those values out below.

My core six values:

Adapted from the works of Russ Harris, 2010, and WR Miller, et. al., 2001.

The Wheel of Life

The Wheel of Life is a way to graphically represent your whole life at this moment. The 8 sections represent important areas of life that are pertinent to most people.

Before addressing your satisfaction with each of these areas, rank them in terms of importance to you at this point in your life. Again, this is not about how satisfied you are in this moment with each area (you can feel an area is very important but be unsatisfied or not prioritize it at this moment). Please rank each of the following areas 1 through 8 with 1 being most important). You can only use each number once, no ties or half points!

Your ranking (1-8)

_____ Practice of medicine / work

_____ Family (includes relatives, parents, and children if applicable / excludes partner)

_____ Personal development & growth

_____ Spirituality / religion

_____ Fun and leisure

_____ Relationships (social and intimate including partner if applicable)

_____ Health

_____ Finances

Next, mark your current level of satisfaction in each area by drawing a line to create a new outer edge on the diagram that follows (1=extremely unsatisfied, 10-extremely satisfied). For example, if you feel your health is a 6 out of 10 in terms of satisfaction, you would draw along the #6 arc within that section (see example on following page).

Rate your level of satisfaction as it is at this point in your life. Use the last three to six months as a guide. Also, if you need guidance as to what a section of the wheel encompasses, some sample questions to facilitate your thinking are provided on the page after the wheel (these questions are by no means exhaustive, most important is what each section means to you, with satisfaction defined by you.)

** some prefer to divide "Relationships" into two subcategories – "Intimate Relationships" and "Social Relationships" if these scores differ

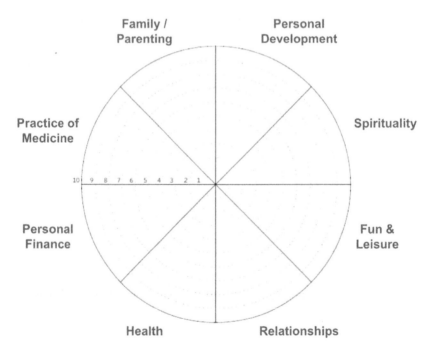

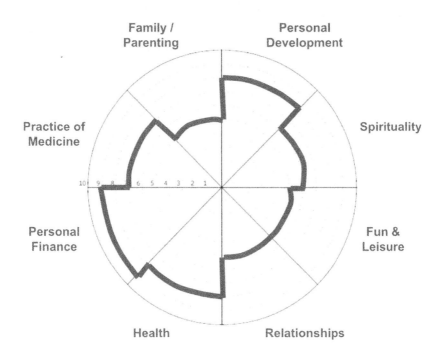

Completed Example

*You do **NOT** need to answer these questions individually. These are simply some questions to help you reflect on and rate your satisfaction in each area on the Wheel of Life.*

Practice of Medicine

Are you able to enjoy your work, colleagues, and patients despite the pressures of daily practice?

Are you living your values as a professional?

Do you continue to be challenged to grow?

Are you fully able to use your knowledge and skills?

Family and Parenting (refers to relationships that you are born into such as parents, siblings, your own children)

Are you satisfied with the level of contact with your family?

Do your family relationships feel open and healthy?

Are you satisfied with your contribution to your family?

Personal Development / Growth

Do you engage in activities and learning that grow and expand you?

Do you have clear and highly-motivating goals for your life?

Do you feel engaged and in control of the unfolding story of your life?

Spirituality

Do you know what you stand for as a human being?

Do you have a deep meaning or motivation for your life?

Do you feel connected to the environment/planet/others in a real way?

Fun & Leisure

Do you regularly take the time you need to experience play, adventure, and leisure?

Do you know what activities renew you make you feel alive?

Do you laugh a lot?

Do you create enough space to relax and enjoy yourself and others?

Relationships (refers to relationships that you are not born into, i.e, partners and friends)
Do you have meaningful experiences with others?
Are you satisfied with what you put into your relationships, and what you get in return?
Do have trust and openness in your relationships? Can you express yourself?
Do your social / intimate relationships support your growth?

Health

Are you satisfied with your level of vitality and physical well-being?
Do you approach your health in a proactive and generative way?
Are you satisfied with your fitness level and your ability to use your body?
Do you have the systems and support structures in place to approach your health with consistency?

Finances

Do you feel that you are managing your finances well?
Are you satisfied with how you use your money?
Do your choices feel sustainable in the big picture?

Made in the USA
Middletown, DE
05 October 2023

40327241R00099